The ADD / ADHD Revolution

The ADD / ADHD Revolution

Treatments That Work

LaVonne & Rick Kirkpatrick

iUniverse, Inc.

New York Lincoln Shanghai

The ADD / ADHD Revolution
Treatments That Work

iUniverse books may be ordered through booksellers or by contacting:

iUniverse
2021 Pine Lake Road, Suite 100
Lincoln, NE 68512
www.iuniverse.com
1-800-Authors (1-800-288-4677)

This book is intended for educational purposes only. Its purpose is to inform about various treatments that others have used for ADHD, as well as to provide evidence currently available regarding the effectiveness of these treatment options. We are not recommending any of these treatments or attempting to give any medical advice. The information in this book is not intended to diagnose, treat, prevent, or cure any disease, including ADHD or in anyway replace the services of a qualified health care professional. We strongly recommend consulting your doctor before using any of these treatments. If your doctor is not aware of what you are doing, he or she will not be fully able to assess the situation and make the appropriate recommendations. Neither the authors nor the publisher shall be liable or responsible for any loss, injury, or damage allegedly arising from any information or suggestion in this book.

ISBN-13: 978-0-595-36935-5 (pbk)
ISBN-13: 978-0-595-81346-9 (ebk)
ISBN-10: 0-595-36935-9 (pbk)
ISBN-10: 0-595-81346-1 (ebk)

Printed in the United States of America

Contents

Introduction

When you picked up this book what were you thinking? Is this just another book on attention deficit disorder and attention deficient hyperactivity disorder? Although countless books and articles have been written on ADD and ADHD, this book takes a unique approach by providing vital information on a wide-range of treatment options.

This book is intended as a guidebook for parents who are looking for possible alternatives and/or additions to medication. The information given in this book has but one purpose: to educate you on the various ADD/ADHD treatments that are presently available. Our goal is to provide you with a comprehensive inventory of these options. No one knows your child better than you do. Therefore, we have researched numerous treatments and our intent is to help you wade through the confusion so you can form your own opinions and make your own treatment choices for your child.

The reality, however, is that although we have made every effort to present this information as simply and objectively as possible, there is no absolute truth to which everyone will agree. Various researchers will come to different conclusions looking at the same research data. Physicians will differ in treatment recommendations while looking at the same test results. Dietitians cannot come to an agreement as to which, if any, vitamins someone should be taking on a daily basis in order to stay healthy.

To make matters even more difficult, not all treatments work equally well for everyone. Just as one medication may be the miracle cure for one person, that same medication may not be helpful at all for another. In fact, it may make the situation worse. Therefore, it becomes a matter of probabilities. You ask: Which ADD/ADHD treatments will have the best chance of working for my child? Ultimately, you will have to make your own choices. The good news is that this book should be a valuable resource for you in that process.

As you read this book, keep in mind that it is focused on giving you information about approaches used in the treatment of ADD/ADHD for children. While treating adults is not the focus, these treatment options are definitely not limited to children. Indeed, most of these treatments may very well be as effective with adults.

This book was designed to answer the many other questions we all have when looking at treating ADD/ADHD. In an effort to gain answers, most of the chapters have been formatted around the following questions:

- What is this treatment option?

- How does the treatment work?

- Who provides this kind of treatment?

- What cost is involved?

- What research has been conducted?

- What is the timeframe or when can results be anticipated?

- What are the pros and cons of its use?

- Where can I get more information? (recommended books, websites, and other resources for more in-depth study)

- What contact information is available?

While reviewing the various treatment approaches, keep in mind that the best solution for your child may not come in the form of any one single treatment modality. Our experience has been that a combination of several treatments appears to be more effective than using only one. The America Medical Association (AMA) now acknowledges that medication and behavioral therapy are often more effective than using medication alone. Here are some things to consider:

- One treatment modality may very well affect another. It may enhance the effect of the other or work adversely against it. Just as in the case of combining medications and supplements, thought should be given to utilizing any variation of multiple treatments.

- If you start using more than one treatment at the same time, it will be difficult to tell which one is being the most effective. If money, time, or your child's resistance is an issue, then taking it slowly and adding only one treatment at a time may be wise.

- Starting or adding several treatment modalities at once may bring quicker results and perhaps even be more effective in the long run. There are times when getting fast results is much more important than knowing which treatment is working best. You can always decrease the treatments later after the desired improvements are achieved.

- We advise you to talk to your treatment provider regarding other therapies you may be using, or considering, so that you can make well-informed decisions. Please remember your child's physician should always be kept informed.

Before considering any treatment option, it is vitally important for parents to seek the best in evaluation. A single checklist or brief 10-minute discussion is not adequate to diagnose your child. Even for a qualified specialist, ADD/ADHD is not always easy to diagnose. Symptoms such as inattention, restlessness, impulsiveness, and academic difficulties can reflect a variety of childhood disorders. These symptoms may also be caused by any number of other factors such as depression, learning disabilities, receptive and expressive language problems, poor nutrition, lack of sleep, allergies, poor parenting skills, and abuse or neglect. It should also be remembered that there have always been children who learn at different rates and have different learning styles which could be misinterpreted. Therefore, a thorough evaluation by a trained clinician is a critical first step. There are several types of specialists qualified to diagnose ADD/ADHD. Among these professionals are child psychiatrists, child psychologists, neurologists, developmental/behavioral pediatricians, and clinical social workers.

ADD or ADHD

ADD? ADHD? What is the right name for the disorder? While this condition has been known for over 100 years, it has not always been called the same thing.

As a result of studies conducted in the 1970s and 1980s, researchers began to recognize the existence of different types of attention deficit. Even though the different types have major differences, they are more alike than different. Consequently, doctors began to see that the different types are all part of the same major condition.

The American Psychiatric Association publishes the official guidelines for naming and diagnosing mental disorders. This book, which is called the *Diagnostic and Statistical Manual of Mental Disorders* (DSM), is updated regularly as more scientific knowledge is learned. In 1994, when the DSM-IV was published, the name ADD (attention deficit disorder) was "officially" changed to ADHD because of the advances in research.[1]

ADHD is the most common behavioral disorder in children. Professionals who diagnose ADHD use the criteria of the DSM. The DSM-IV-TR, which is the most recent version, classifies the disorder into the following three subtypes:

- Predominantly inattentive

- Predominantly hyperactive/impulsive

- Combined [2]

Some doctors and mental health professionals, however, still continue to use the term ADD. If this is your child's diagnosis, most likely your child has the inattentive type of ADHD. Such an individual is easily distracted and just can't seem to pay attention. Additionally, this child may be forgetful and disorganized, as well as often appearing to be daydreaming. This is definitely not the individual described as "bouncing off the walls" or being "incapable of sitting still."

We acknowledge that ADHD is the term currently being used in diagnosing all subtypes of this disorder. However, we also recognize the many parents, as well as the general public, may be just as comfortable using the term ADD, now considered as outdated in the most recent DSM publication. Therefore, whether your child is primarily inattentive, primarily hyperactive/impulsive, or a combination of the two, for simplification we will use the term ADHD when referring to this disorder throughout the remainder of the book.

"Alternative" Treatments

The term "alternative" is used to describe the various techniques, modalities, and products which are presented as treatment options. Most people tend to use "alternative" when talking about any treatment other than what has traditionally been used. However, you may see other terms, such as complementary, integrative, or Complementary and Alternative Medicine (CAM), associated with these treatment options as you read the literature. Although we call these alternative treatments, we do not see them replacing the more traditional treatments. Rather, we view them as "complementing or being integrated with" traditional treatments.

Final Thoughts

As you read our book, remember that none of the options described are the answer for every child diagnosed with ADHD. No one treatment works equally well for everyone. There is no definite cure for ADHD. However, we believe it is vitally important for parents to educate themselves on the possible treatment options. This resource book provides a starting point for concerned parents to investigate what is available and to make informed decisions.

Remember that you, like many other parents, are searching for information in order to help your child. We support your efforts in seeking to learn about everything you can which might possibly help your ADHD child. The more information you have, the better off both you and your child will be. Our desire is for this book to positively impact the lives of both ADHD children and their families.

1

Being an Informed Parent

Prevalence and Consequences

Approximately three to five percent of the school-aged population in the United States is thought to have ADHD, although some experts would place the percentage at an even higher rate. Being diagnosed as having ADHD increases the likelihood of having several other problems as well. Individuals with ADHD are at risk for such conditions as oppositional defiant disorder, conduct disorder, learning disabilities, anxiety, and depression. This phenomenon of coexisting conditions is referred to as comorbidity.[1]

Children with ADHD have been identified in every country in which ADHD has been studied. While it has long been thought that ADHD is more common in boys than girls, recent research indicates that the actual numbers may be almost equal.[2] Boys with ADHD are typically more aggressive than girls. Therefore, girls are often older than boys by the time they are diagnosed and they are less likely to be referred for treatment.[3]

As a parent, you may have received a phone call or a series of phone calls from your child's teacher voicing her concern that your child is not paying attention, can't seem to sit still, and/or is not learning in the classroom setting. Perhaps you have also had several face-to-face conferences with your child's teacher. She may have suggested that you see your doctor to inquire about using stimulant medication to help your child in focusing and being more attentive. Or, perhaps you yourself are wondering if your child may have ADHD because of significant problems at school or at home. If you have experienced one or more of these scenarios, this book is designed to be a valuable resource as you begin to seek help for your child.

ADHD is far from a benign disorder. For those who have it, it can cause devastating problems. According to the International Consensus Statement on ADHD (January 2002), studies suggest that those who have this disorder are far more likely than the general population to drop out of school (32-40%), to graduate rarely from college (5-10%), to have few or no friends (50-70%), to under perform at work (70-80%), to engage in antisocial activities (40-50%), and to use tobacco or illegal drugs more than the normal population. In addition, children growing up with ADHD are more likely to become pregnant as a teenager (40%), experience sexually transmitted diseases (16%), to speed excessively and be involved in multiple car accidents (20-30%), and to experience depression (20-30%), and personality disorders (18-25%) as adults.[4]

Despite these serious consequences, studies point out that less than half of those with the disorder are receiving treatment. As a parent of an ADHD child, you need to become an "expert" on this topic. No doubt you are well aware of how challenging your job can be; you definitely want to obtain the very best possible treatment for your child. Since you are responsible for investing your family's time, money, and energy wisely, being an informed parent is a top priority.

Remember, knowledge is power. Through your knowledge of ADHD and your familiarity with the needs of your child, you can better coordinate treatment by health professionals, communicate with educators, and be an advocate for your child to ensure that the best possible programs are in place to help your child to succeed.

How ADHD can best be treated is a matter of intense debate. Typically, current treatments involve medication, behavioral therapy, or both. Since these traditional treatments are extensively used and so well known, we will not spend much time on them. There is ample information on these subjects from a number of other sources and this book's intent is to provide you with information on some of the lesser known treatments. However, if you are just now starting to learn about all of the various treatments for ADHD, you may find the following overviews on medications and behavioral therapy helpful.

Medications

If you are considering medication for your child, he or she should first undergo a thorough, comprehensive assessment to clarify the diagnosis and to identify any other medical, psychological, or learning problems which may be present. Next a treatment plan should be developed in consultation with your physician or other medical/mental health professional. In this planning stage all parties (child, family and medical professional) should work as a team to consider the various options available for treatment.

At the beginning of the medication trial, careful monitoring is essential. If the first medication is not helpful or produces negative side effects, the prescribing professional will need to adjust the dosage or timing, or both. If the response is not positive after adjustments are made, another medication may need to be tried.

According to the New Treatment Guidelines for ADHD from the American Academy of Pediatrics, children may respond favorably to one stimulant, but not another. As a result, physicians should not switch to a non-stimulant medication for treating ADHD until the child has been tested on at least two or three different stimulants across a full range of doses without showing any significantly positive response.[5]

Since doctors are trained to diagnose and label diseases, your doctor may likely recommend or prescribe drugs to relieve your child's ADHD symptoms. Stimulant medications are the most commonly prescribed. The most popular ones are Ritalin, Methylin, Adderall, Dexedrine, Cylert, and Concerta. Antidepressants, such as Desipramine, Imipramine, and Wellbutrin, may be prescribed for children who don't respond to stimulant medications or who have other psychiatric problems. A third group of drugs sometimes prescribed for ADHD children are anti-hypertensive, or blood pressure lowering drugs, such as Clonidine or Tenex.[6]

With over 150 controlled, double-blind studies of stimulant use in children with ADHD, the findings concerning medication treatments are well documented. However, as a discerning parent you need to examine both the pros and cons of giving your child stimulant medication.

There are several positive aspects of using stimulant medications. Among these are the following:

- These medications are relatively easy to use and they work quickly. Therefore, you will know in a short period of time whether they are going to help or not. Short-acting preparations generally are effective for about four hours. Longer-acting newer preparations are more variable with some lasting up to 10 or 12 hours. Since there can be wide individual variation, however, the exact lasting effect of the medication will only become known once the medication is tried.

- There is evidence that stimulant medications improve both behavior and school performance.

- They are relatively inexpensive.

- Stimulants have been used as a treatment for many years, so doctors have considerable experience in prescribing them.

- Medication may provide immediate relief for a child who is about to be expelled from school or whose family is experiencing a "melt-down" under the strain of the situation.[7]

Current evidence indicates that stimulant medications are safe and well tolerated by most children. A majority of side effects occur early in the treatment, appear short-lived, and can usually be successfully managed through adjusting the dosage or by changing the medication. Medication can often help a multi-modal (combination) treatment program be more effective. Although no adverse effects of long-term use of stimulant medications are currently known, there is a definite need for long-term safety studies.[8]

Stimulant medications, however, are not without their negative aspects. Some of these concerns are as follows:

- About 20 to 30% of children with ADHD do not respond to stimulant medication.

- Children's appetites may be suppressed by stimulants, thereby initially affecting their growth and normal weight gain.

- A few children complain of frequent stomach aches and/or headaches while taking stimulant medication.

- Some children may be especially difficult to manage later in the day or evening when the medication has worn off.

- Children on stimulants may also have trouble falling asleep.

- A very small percentage of children on stimulant medication develop latent tics. These involuntary movements may include eye blinking, shrugging, and/or clearing of the throat. It is estimated that 7% of children with ADHD have tics or Tourette's syndrome, a chronic disorder that involves vocal and motor tics, while 60% of children with Tourette's have ADHD. Although recent research indicates that the development of Tourette's in children with ADHD is not related to stimulant medication, a cautious approach to using stimulants is recommended if there is a family history of Tourette's or tics.[9]

- Some children experience embarrassment if they have to get their medication from the nurse during the school day.

Maximizing the Benefits of Stimulant Medication Treatment

Children treated in research studies often do better than children treated with the same medication by their family physicians. You may be wondering why this is the case. One of the primary reasons is that children treated in community settings may often be maintained on doses that are not sufficient to provide maximal benefit. Even though the recently published treatment guidelines by the American Academy of Pediatrics recommend systematic monitoring of children's responses to a full range of stimulant medication dosages, the reality is that this recommendation has often been neglected in community practice settings.[10]

In most research studies, such as the Multimodal Treatment Study (MTA), participants are tested on several different doses of stimulant medication and a placebo, with systematic monitoring of the children's responses occurring after each treatment to find the most effective treatment. Additionally, ongoing treatment effectiveness may be monitored with frequent follow-up visits and telephone contacts with children's teachers and parents.

Once an initial optimal dosage is found, it is important to note that adjustments in dosages will very likely be required to sustain maximum treatment benefits over time. For example, in the MTA study, only 17% of the children continued on the same medication and dosage level throughout the entire 13-month maintenance period. All of the other participants had at least one change in drug or dosage for that time period. While the average number of changes required for each child was two, some children had as many as 10 adjustments. Of the total number of changes implemented over the 13-month period, 62% involved increasing dosages, 31% involved decreasing dosages and only 7% involved changing medications completely.[11]

In contrast, ongoing monitoring of a medication's effectiveness is typically far less intensive in a community setting. This can result in a less than optimal benefit to your child. It is also not uncommon for family physicians to discontinue the initial stimulant medication, if unsuccessful, and to switch to another class of medication, such as anti-depressants, before trying other stimulants.

As a parent who may be considering stimulant medication, there are several points you should keep in mind in order for your child to receive the optimal benefit from your choice. Here are several suggestions:

1. It is important that your child be tested on a full range of doses when beginning medication treatment.

    •   Even though the first dose may produce positive results, it may not be the best dose to maximize your child's functioning.

    •   Optimal dosages are not weight dependent, so it is impossible to predict ahead of time what the most effective stimulant or best dosage will be.

2. Insist on a systematic procedure for monitoring the effectiveness of the different dosages being tested.

    •   Your child's academic functioning, social skills, and willingness/ability to follow rules at home and at school all need monitoring. A systematic procedure for evaluating side effects should also be implemented.

    •   Routinely receiving direct and detailed feedback from your child's teachers is vital. Informally hearing that he or she is "doing better" is not sufficient.

3. If the first stimulant medication tested does not produce positive results, it is recommended that two or three other stimulants be tried in varying dosages before non-stimulant medications be considered, or combining other medications with a stimulant.

    •   A recent report shows that almost 25% of children who take stimulant medication are also taking a second medication. Since the safety and effectiveness of combined pharmacotherapy for ADHD children is very limited, it is recommended that you proceed with caution if you receive such a recommendation.[12]

Behavioral Therapy

Children with ADHD often benefit greatly from behavioral therapy or counseling, which may be provided by a psychiatrist, psychologist, social worker, licensed professional counselor, marriage and family therapist, or other mental health care professional. Psychotherapy, behavioral therapy, family therapy, social skills training, parenting skills training, and support groups are among the treatment options that are available to you.[13]

Through psychotherapy, older children and adults with ADHD talk about various issues that are bothering them and explore negative behavioral patterns they have been exhibiting. In this way, they learn more effective ways to deal with their symptoms. Some individuals with ADHD may also have coexisting conditions, such as depression or anxiety disorder. In these cases of comorbidity, counseling therapies may help both the coexisting problem as well as the ADHD.

Behavioral therapy helps both teachers and parents learn strategies for dealing with the behavior of ADHD children. Some of these contingency management procedures include token reward systems and timeouts. Behavior modification utilizing contingency management strategies has proven especially beneficial for individuals with ADHD.

Since children with ADHD are not the only ones affected by this condition, family therapy may assist both parents and siblings to deal with the stress of living with an ADHD child. Parents, often feeling hopeless and alone, are depressed and frustrated with the challenge of raising a child with ADHD. Additionally, siblings are significantly affected and should be educated about ADHD. It is important to assure younger brothers or sisters that ADHD is not a transmittable disease is order to prevent fear or avoidance of the ADHD brother or sister. Older siblings may also need assistance in understanding the symptoms of ADHD and how to help their younger ADHD sibling. Being more knowledgeable will help them to deal with unpleasant situations and to avoid embarrassment, especially in front of their peers.[14]

Social skills training can help children learn appropriate social behaviors. Most children with ADHD have great difficulty in developing and maintaining peer relationships. ADHD symptoms such as inattentiveness or impulsivity can certainly cause the child to have difficulty displaying the appropriate behaviors. However, even more problematic is that the child often does not learn the appropriate behaviors or the social cues that guide all of us in our social relationships. Sometimes it is necessary to relearn what is appropriate as well as to pay attention to social cues. For many children with ADHD, the ability to read body language is a concept they do not comprehend.

Training in parenting skills can assist the parents in developing ways to understand and guide their child's behavior. For example, the American Academy of Pediatrics recommends the following three basic principles: (1) setting clear and specific rules, (2) providing consistent consequences for inappropriate behavior and positive rewards for appropriate behavior, and (3) using these rewards and consequences on a regular and long-term basis.[15] Structure is also vital for an ADHD child. These children, in particular, need a stable, daily routine and clear organization in the home. Even a simple routine which creates a designated place for items such as backpacks and toys will save the child and the parent a great deal of frustration.

Support groups offer ADHD children and their parents and families a network of social support, information, and education. In addition, support groups aid parents in feeling less alone, allowing them to share their mistakes, frustrations, and successes with others in similar situations.

Children and Adults with Attention-Deficit/Hyperactivity Disorder (CHADD), with chapters and satellites located in more than 225 communities across the country, is one of the more well known organizations serving individuals with ADHD. Local CHADD groups offer various activities which may include the following: (1) support groups, (2) community resource information, (3) monthly meetings on topics of interest, (4) outreach programs, and (5) networking opportunities with other adults, parents, and professionals interested in ADHD.[16]

Generally, the best results occur when a team approach is used, with parents/family, teachers, and therapists or physicians working together. Also, making every effort to work with your child's teachers and referring them to reliable sources of information to assist their efforts with your child in the classroom are extremely important.

Deciding about Treatment Options

If you ask your child's teachers or physician for their advice regarding medication, don't be surprised if they encourage the idea of taking it. For one thing, they both have the most familiarity with medication. Teachers are looking for increased manageability of your child in the classroom setting; physicians are adhering to the medical model in which they were trained.

As a parent, however, you will need to make up your own mind regarding medication. You certainly should not have your child take medication if you are not comfortable with the idea. Regardless of your decision, remember that medication is not a magic cure.

As voiced in the introductory chapter, there is no definite cure for ADHD. No one treatment works equally well for everyone. You, as a parent, need to educate yourself on the wide range of possible interventions available. For best results, it is recommended that the treatment of ADHD be comprehensive.

Regardless of the type of intervention(s) or treatment(s) your child is receiving, it is essential that a thorough monitoring plan be in place. Without careful monitoring of ongoing treatment effectiveness, information that is necessary to determine when adjustments may be needed will not be available. As a result, your child may receive less than the maximum benefits from any treatment option.

Dr. David Rabiner, research psychologist at the Center for Child and Family Policy at Duke University, has developed a relatively simple monitoring system which provides an example of how to gather and interpret important information from your child's teachers. It is available at no cost (www. helpforadd.com/monitor.htm).

Examining New Treatments

There are some basic guidelines for evaluating any new treatments, whether these treatments are among those options described in this book or others you may hear or read about from other sources. Be skeptical of any new treatment or product that does the following:

- Makes exaggerated or overstated claims
- Is being touted as a "miracle" treatment or as a "truly amazing break-through"
- Claims to treat virtually all conditions or ailments (The more grandiose the claim, the less likely it is that there is any real merit to it.)
- Claims it is being unfairly attacked by the medical establishment

Research Information

There are basically two ways in which treatment options are evaluated. They are (1) standard scientific procedure and (2) limited case studies or testimonials. Carefully controlled scientific studies involve specific criteria such as utilizing large numbers of subjects, replicating studies, randomly assigning individuals to treatment groups, implementing double-blind procedures, and employing a placebo-control.

With the scientific approach, a relatively large number of subjects or participants are used to allow the researchers to be comfortable with the "strength" of their findings. These studies are repeated over time by various research teams in order to conclude that a specific treatment helps a specific problem. By randomly assigning participants to treatment groups, researchers deal with the possibility that there may have been group differences that existed prior to when treatment began that could account for the differences after treatment, rather than the differences being attributed to the treatment itself.

In a "double-blind" study, neither the researcher nor the participant is aware of (blind to) the nature of the treatment the participant is receiving. Double blind trials are thought to produce more objective results since the expectations of the researcher and the participant about the treatment do not affect the outcome.

If the double-blind study is "placebo-controlled," a fake treatment (placebo) is given to one group of participants while the treatment (such as medication) being tested is given to another group. The "placebo effect" is a phenomenon in which a fake treatment can sometimes improve a patient's condition simply because the patient expects that it will be beneficial. To separate out this factor and some other variables from a treatment's true benefits, placebo-controlled studies are often used. If patients on the new treatment fared significantly better than those who took the placebo, the results will help support the conclusion that the treatment is effective.

With limited case studies and testimonials, which is the second way of evaluating treatment options, one does not have the solid evidence resulting from controlled studies. Therefore, within the medical and scientific communities, individuals often voice their concern over the lack of carefully controlled scientific studies, as described previously, for many of the treatment options we will be discussing in this book. In fact, several of these treatment options may be supported only by testimonials and case studies from health care providers and their patients with almost no or very limited research findings to substantiate their claims.

Remember, however, that a treatment that is supported only in this manner is not necessarily an ineffective treatment. Keep in mind that there may be other factors to help explain the lack of scientific study for some of these treatments. Indeed, some of these treatments may not readily lend themselves to such scientific controls. For example, since parents tend to choose whether their child will receive a treatment and pay for its cost, the reality of randomly assigning subjects to treatment groups is often quite impractical. Since research studies are expensive, funding such studies becomes a challenge. Also, few researchers choose to study treatments for ADHD that are not patentable, which is the case for many natural products. Another factor to consider is whether or not a treatment is fairly new. If that is the case, there may not have been time for extensive research to have been conducted. Finally, to keep everything in perspective, consider the case of heart by-pass surgery. Most of us know someone who has successfully undergone this procedure. However, how many double-blind placebo controlled studies were conducted using this treatment option? Although the answer is none, you would not discount its effectiveness.

We do recognize the value of carefully controlled scientific studies. Certainly more research studies on any treatment would be welcomed. As we emphasized in the introductory chapter, our purpose is to provide you with pertinent information on every option covered in this book to help you draw your own conclusions and make your own decisions based on the information currently available.

Note:

A glossary of the more common research terms and assessments or rating scales mentioned in the research section of each chapter is included at the end of this book. This is done in an effort to simplify the reading of these chapters while providing the necessary information for a more in-depth understanding of the research if needed.

2

EEG Neurofeedback

* Professional Provider Systems

* Play Attention

* S.M.A.R.T. BrainGames

Electroencephalogram (EEG) neurofeedback training is a painless, drug-free, and non-invasive procedure. It is a form of biofeedback where the individual's brainwaves, also called EEG, are used. While there are several types of EEG biofeedback, for clarification purposes it is important to note that any of these types may be called by a number of different names. These names are EEG neurobiofeedback, EEG biofeedback, neurofeedback, neurobiofeedback, and brainwave training. For clarity, EEG biofeedback is any feedback from a physiological system including cardio pulmonary, respiratory, etc. EEG neurofeedback is a highly specialized form of biofeedback that solely monitors brainwave signals.

One way of looking at the various types of EEG neurobiofeedback is by who provides the training. From this perspective, there are three types of systems that are available at the present time. One type is what we will refer to as the "Professional Provider System." This type of training is primarily provided in a professional's office and usually done by someone who has had extensive training in EEG neurofeedback as well as in the medical, psychological, or educational fields. This is what might be considered the traditional method that has been practiced for a number of years.

Recently, variations of this method have been developed and are presently on the market. The second type of system we will look at is a home-based system called Play Attention®. With this system, the child's parent usually provides all the training at home under the professional supervision of Play Attention's educational support staff. This method also adds cognitive skill training and behavioral shaping as part of the training modality.

The third type of system is called S.M.A.R.T. (Self Mastery and Regulation Training) BrainGames™. It is a system where a professional provider does some of the training in his or her office while the parent does the majority of the training at home.

There are several theories that may explain why EEG neurofeedback is effective. In traditional EEG neurofeedback, an attempt is made to change brainwave patterns that may produce desired physical outcomes. Others do not think the brainwaves change at all, but that the EEG neurofeedback mainly sets the stage for new learning to take place. Since this book is geared toward simplifying fairly complex treatments, we will not go into various theories but will give you one theory that will help you to understand EEG neurofeedback from the traditional view.

From this standpoint, EEG neurofeedback can be seen as a form of operant conditioning. Just as children will tend to do more of those behaviors for which they are rewarded, the brain will also start doing more of those behaviors for which it is rewarded. Since the brain is pliable and capable of learning new behaviors throughout life, it can learn new brainwave patterns and, over time, reproduce them on its own without the need for further brainwave training. These new brainwave patterns are associated with improved functioning, allowing the brain to better control itself, and therefore, resulting in an improvement for a broad range of conditions including ADHD and its related symptoms.

Generally, it is theorized that individuals with ADHD have an excess of slower brainwaves as compared to the general population. These brainwaves are called alpha and theta. They are associated with a brain that has some trouble regulating itself. Some children with ADHD also have an excess of fast brainwaves. These brainwaves are called high beta and are associated with tension and anxiety. As one might expect, these excessive brainwaves result in less than optimal functioning of the brain and can produce many symptoms associated with ADHD. The goal of traditional EEG neurofeedback is to reduce the excessive brainwaves and increase the brainwaves associated with good brain regulation. These good brain waves are called SMR and low beta.

One way of looking at this brain regulation is that it is simply strength and flexibility training for the brain. It exercises the brain in being flexible so that it can shift to producing more "good" brainwaves and fewer "bad" brainwaves. This exercising also builds up strength so that the brain can continue producing the "good" brainwave patterns even after the training sessions are over.

All three of the EEG neurofeedback methods use one or more sensors that are placed on the scalp where they pick up the brainwave activity and send it to a computer. This brainwave signal is then processed and turned into a visual display on a screen. This display is usually in the form of some sort of computer video game. The rewards that the individual receives while playing the games are visual, auditory, and sometimes tactile such as vibration. (It is important to note that the sensors only pick up electrical activity and do not shock or conduct any electrical current to the child.)

The video game shows the individual what the brain is doing, and the person controls the game with his/her brain; no joystick is used except with S.M.A.R.T. BrainGames. Generally speaking, the more the brain produces the desired frequency, the better the game works and rewards the individual. Gradually, the brain responds to the cues that it is being given, and over time, it learns to produce the improved brainwave patterns on its own. These new patterns are directly associated with the brain's ability to function better, causing enhanced self-regulation and improved behaviors.

Professional Provider Systems

This section describes clinical EEG biofeedback that is provided by professionals. As such, this training can be used to treat a broad range of problem areas and not simply attention-related issues that the home-based units are designed to do.

Names:

EEG Neurofeedback
EEG Biofeedback
Neurofeedback
Neurobiofeedback
Brainwave Training

This form of treatment may be referred to by any of the above mentioned names. There is no agreed upon name which all providers of this treatment use and no single company providing these systems that has the legal rights to their use and protocols.

What it is:

The primary difference that separates this type of EEG neurofeedback from the others is the level of involvement that the EEG neurofeedback provider offers. The provider does the initial assessment, selection of protocols, and is present during the treatment to make ongoing assessments and adjustments to the program. The professional provider is also there to answer all questions and to reassess the situation as training progresses.

How it works:

The training is usually done in the EEG neurofeedback provider's office as the child sits in a comfortable chair. After an initial assessment, the provider makes the decision as to where on the scalp the sensors need to be placed to achieve the desired outcome. The provider then individually places the sensors and assures that a good contact is made with a paste or saline solution. Once the brainwave frequencies are picked up and sent to the computer, they are amplified and analyzed by the provider. At this point the provider decides which frequencies need to be suppressed and which ones need to be encouraged for optimal brain functioning. During the session the provider monitors the frequencies and the child's immediate response, making appropriate changes to these frequencies and/or electrode placements as needed.

Training sessions:

Training times usually last from 30-45 minutes, with a little time added before and after each session for evaluation and cleanup. The sessions are usually conducted two or three times per week in the provider's office.

Many children will need between 20-40 sessions and some may need 40-60 sessions or more to complete the training. For a child with ADHD, 40 sessions would be considered reasonable.

Some providers are equipped to provide home training after a set number of sessions in the office. Home training sessions are the same as the ones that are done in the office, except the parent is taught how to use the equipment and the provider monitors the home training and progress. Any needed protocol changes are done either by the client returning periodically to the provider's office or by the provider explaining to the parent what to do.

Providers:

A professional in the behavioral sciences, and/or the health and educational fields, such as a physician, psychologist, or mental health therapist, usually provides EEG neurofeedback services. However, other professionals may obtain the training and provide this service as well. These providers usually receive extensive specialty training in the area of EEG neurofeedback in addition to their professional training.

In choosing a provider, you may want to consider a provider that can address other issues that your child may have as well. While EEG neurofeedback is used for all ADHD related symptoms including hyperactivity, distractibility, impulsively, and inattention, it is also being used for other conditions which frequently occur along with ADHD. Such conditions include sleep problems, Tourette's syndrome, depression, bipolar disorder, seizures, anxiety disorders, conduct disorder, and some learning disabilities. In fact, EEG neurofeedback is being used for many conditions in which the brain is not working as well as it might. The research and anecdotal evidence vary depending upon the condition treated.

There is a certification in EEG neurofeedback provided by the Biofeedback Certification Institute of America (BCIA). Finding a provider with this certification may be helpful in choosing a provider. However, in most states, it is not required that a provider has this certification and there are good EEG neurofeedback providers who offer this training without it. Referrals from others who have received this training from the provider and the years of experience this professional has in providing the service should also be factors in your selection process.

Cost:

The cost of services varies depending upon who is doing the training. Most providers charge a comparable amount to what their profession usually charges. If a psychologist provides the training, he/she usually charges from $75 to $100 a session, while a professional educator may charge from $50 to $100. Some individuals provide this service for as little as $50 per session. The cost of 40 sessions would ordinarily range from $2,000 to $4,000. Keep in mind, however, it does not mean that the more one is charged the better the treatment.

Additionally, there is usually a charge for an assessment which is separate from the treatment sessions. These charges vary depending upon who is doing the assessment, the test given, and the duration of the assessment. Assessment costs might run anywhere from $150 to $400.

In regard to insurance, more progressive medical plans may cover EEG neurofeedback for various conditions. However, many medical plans do not cover this cost. Your specific coverage questions will need to be addressed to your insurance company.

Research:

Neurofeedback training is based upon more than thirty years of research. Yet, within the medical and scientific communities, viewpoints differ widely concerning the usefulness of neurofeedback treatment for ADHD. At one extreme are those who focus on the lack of specific scientific data documenting the effectiveness of this approach. On the other end of the continuum are researchers and practitioners who argue that several published studies clearly establish the value and usefulness of this treatment.

Neurofeedback vs. Stimulant Medication: Matched Treatment Groups

In one study EEG biofeedback was compared to psychostimulant medication.[1] There were 46 participants (37 boys, 9 girls) who were between 8 and 21 years of age and had IQs between 80 and 120. The Test of Variables of Attention (TOVA) was administered before and after treatment.

After 20 treatment sessions completed over a period of four to seven weeks, the EEG biofeedback treatment group improved significantly on all four areas of the TOVA. In addition, reports from parents and teachers supported the TOVA results. The medication group also improved in all four TOVA areas.

There was no significant difference between the groups in the degree of improvement shown. Therefore, the researchers concluded that EEG biofeedback is an effective alternative to stimulants and may be preferred in cases where medication is not effective or only partially effective, has adverse side effects, or where compliance with taking medication is low.

Neurofeedback vs. Control Group Study

Another study randomly assigned 18 children (ages 5 to 15) to either a neurofeedback treatment or a wait-list control group.[2] None of the children were on medication. The neurofeedback group received 40 sessions, two per week, extending over six months.

All 18 children were assessed before and after treatment on various measures including intellectual functioning and parental behavioral reports of inattentiveness, hyperactivity, aggression, and defiant behaviors. Compared with the control group, the neurofeedback group demonstrated significant reductions in inattentive behaviors as well as showing significant increases in scores on an intelligence test.

Neurofeedback as Part of Comprehensive Treatment Model

More recently, a larger study was conducted involving 100 children ranging in age from 6 to 19.[3] None of the 83 boys and 17 girls had a history of prior treatment for ADHD.

Parents of 51 participants chose to include neurofeedback as part of their child's comprehensive treatment program, along with medication, counseling, and academic support. The other 49 parents chose not to include the neurofeedback component. Neurofeedback sessions lasting 30 to 40 minutes were conducted on a weekly basis.

The two groups of children did not differ in age, gender, IQ, or socioeconomic status. Parent and teacher ratings regarding ADHD symptoms and participants' scores on the Test of Variables of Attention (TOVA), on the Attention Deficit Disorders Evaluation Scale (ADDES), and on the QEEG scan were equivalent prior to the treatment.

After one year of treatments, the children were tested twice, once when they were still on medication and a second time after they had been off medication for one week. Significant improvement was noted in both groups on the TOVA and ADDES when participants were tested while using Ritalin. In contrast, only those in the neurofeedback treatment group sustained those gains when the medication was discontinued.

Parents and teachers of children in the neurofeedback group also reported fewer inattentive, hyperactive, and impulsive behaviors both at home and at school after one week without medication. Additionally, children whose parents consistently used effective reinforcement strategies displayed fewer ADHD symptoms.

These findings support comprehensive treatment models that include parent counseling and EEG biofeedback, in addition to stimulant therapy (medication). The researchers report the only type of behavior therapy associated with sustained improvement of core ADHD symptoms in the absence of medication has been EEG biofeedback. One of the implications is that the benefits of neurofeedback are retained when children are not receiving treatment.

German Study: Neurofeedback vs. Stimulant Medication

Another recent study in Germany compared the effects of a 12-week neurofeedback program with stimulant medication. Participants were 34 children, ages 8 through 12.[4] The 22 participants (21 boys, 1 girl) in the neurofeedback group did not receive any medication during the entire study.

The 12 participants (12 boys) in the stimulant medication group were administered Ritalin, three times daily on school days. Individual dosages varied between 10 and 60 mg per day. EEG neurofeedback training consisted of three 30-60 minute training sessions per week conducted on weekday afternoons.

There were no pretreatment differences between the groups on any of the following assessment measures: TOVA, Attention Endurance Test, German versions of the IOWA-Conners' Behavior Rating Scale and the Wechsler Intelligence Scale for Children-Revised (WISC-R).

Post-treatment results reported significant improvements were shown for both groups on all assessment measures except one. Unlike some other studies there were no significant improvements on the intelligence scales for either the neurofeedback or medication group.

Discussion

A limitation in all the above studies is the lack of follow-up for any sustained time period after treatment ended for the children participating in these studies. Because of this limitation, it is not clear whether improvements associated with neurofeedback continued for any significant period after the training concluded.

In the CHADD (Children and Adults with Attention-Deficit/Hyperactivity Disorder) Fact Sheet #6, it is reported that EEG biofeedback treatment has been used for over 25 years and that many parents have reported this treatment option as "extremely helpful" for their child.[5] The fact sheet also acknowledges that there have been several published studies of neurofeedback treatment that have shown promising results. However, CHADD cautions that controlled randomized trials need to be conducted before more definitive conclusions regarding the effectiveness of EEG biofeedback can be reached.

Today's debate about neurofeedback is basically no different from what was occurring 10 or 15 years ago. While several research teams have demonstrated the effectiveness of neurofeedback for ADHD, uncertainty regarding its effectiveness will no doubt continue until more large-scale studies which provide for the necessary scientific controls are conducted. Although more research is still necessary, there have been numerous case study reports and several promising investigations citing positive results in the use of neurofeedback treatments.

Results:

EEG training is a learning process, and therefore results are seen gradually over time. You will usually observe changes in 5 to 10 sessions. Individual results will vary, depending upon age and severity of symptoms. If the child has a number of symptoms, it is common that some symptoms start improving before others.

Once learning is consolidated, the benefits appear to be permanent in most cases. The total number of sessions that it takes to make the changes permanent is hard to estimate but is usually around 20 to 40. Many professionals will taper off the sessions toward the end of the training to ensure that the child maintains the improvements as the sessions become farther and farther apart.

As the research in this chapter shows, EEG neurofeedback does not work for everyone. There is no guarantee that your child will be helped at all. However, the research does show that there is a high probability that at least some of the symptoms of ADHD will be substantially reduced.

Pros & cons

Cautions: No permanent adverse side effects of the training have been documented when a trained professional has provided the service. However, there can be temporary symptoms, such as headaches, which are usually remedied through adjustments in training protocols. If children are on medications, the dosage may need to be reduced or eliminated as the training progresses. Therefore it is necessary for a physician to be kept informed regarding the child's condition so that he/she does not become overmedicated.

Time: Since each session can take up to an hour and is usually done two or three times per week, time can be an issue as well. Also, scheduling a fairly large number of sessions adds to the time commitment. However, finding a provider who does home training can assist with reducing the time commitment.

Convenience: While the number of EEG neurofeedback providers is growing, their numbers are still not large. It may be difficult to find a provider near you, thereby making it inconvenient to obtain the training. Keep in mind that many providers are willing to work with you in helping obtain the training in a more convenient manner. When a client has to drive a long way, some providers are willing to work with their clients to provide marathon sessions done on weekends only. Also, home training may be a possibility when distance is an issue.

Other: One of the major advantages of working with a professional in the behavioral or medical sciences who provides EEG biofeedback services is that these individuals can also address other conditions that often occur along with ADHD.

Recommended reading and websites:

ADD: The 20-Hour Solution
Training Minds to Concentrate and Self-Regulate Naturally without Medication
Authors: Mark Steinberg, Ph. D. & Siegfried Othmer, Ph.D.
Robert D. Reed Publishers Copyright 2004
This is a comprehensive book that explains all aspects of EEG biofeedback in easy to understand terms. It talks about what ADD really is and how EEG biofeedback works for this condition. It also includes a list of EEG biofeedback providers worldwide.

Getting Rid of Ritalin: How Neurofeedback Can Successfully Treat Attention Deficit Disorder without Drugs
Authors: Robert W. Hill, Ph.D. & Edwardo Castro, M.D.
Hampton Roads Publishing Company, Inc. Copyright 2002
This book talks about ADD and various factors which can affect this disorder. These factors range from nutritional concerns and supplements to toxic sub-

stances and parenting skills. It also does a very good job describing EEG bio-feedback and how it works. It also includes a list of EEG biofeedback providers worldwide.

The A.D.D. Book: New Understandings, New Approaches to Parenting Your Child
Authors: William Sears, M.D. and Lynda Thompson, Ph.D.
Little Brown and Company Copyright 1998
This book primarily talks about managing ADD without the use of drugs. It talks about helping the ADD child through the use of a variety of interventions such as parenting skills, behavior modification, and nutrition. It is not a book on EGG biofeedback but does have a chapter devoted to this intervention.

Healing ADD: The Breakthrough Program That Allows You to See and Heal the Six Types of Attention Deficit Disorder
Author: Daniel G. Amen, M.D.
Berkley Publishing Group Copyright 2002
The book talks about six types of ADD (Attention Deficit Disorder) and has information on a variety of treatments for ADD in addition to EEG biofeedback. This book does not focus on EEG biofeedback but is very informative for those exploring various treatments for ADD.

A Symphony in the Brain: The Evolution of the New Brain Wave Biofeedback
Author: Jim Robbins
Grove/Atlantic, Inc. Copyright 2001
This book tells the story of the development of EEG biofeedback. It includes case studies, scientific explanations of EEG biofeedback, and personal accounts of its uses. This is a good book for those who want to understand how EEG biofeedback got to be where it is today.

There are other websites with information on EEG biofeedback but the three listed below are among the best available for a parent to gain a simple yet comprehensive understanding of the basics of EEG biofeedback. Each of these websites contains research, case studies, and personal stories. They also have lists of EEG providers and links to other websites for those who want to dig deeper.

www.eegspectrum.com
www.EEGInstitute.com
www.eeginfo.com

Contact information:

To find a provider near you, it is suggested you look on the websites listed in this chapter. Several organizations have a world wide provider list posted on their sites. You can also call one of the organizations to obtain a list of providers. A couple of the books mentioned at the end of this chapter also include a list of providers. (See book descriptions.)

Play Attention

Name:

Play Attention®

What it is:

This system is a pre-calibrated EEG, physiological monitor which cannot be altered (re-calibrated). It is designed to be done in the home under continuous professional supervision via a distance learning program so that minimal training is needed by the parents or the child. Therefore, the necessity of going to a professional's office is eliminated. It also has the addition of Edufeedback®, which is comprised of educational protocols and methodology that are patented and exclusive to Play Attention. The system is designed to combine cognitive skill building tools with EEG biofeedback to help the child be able to better utilize the new skills in his or her class work. Unique Logic & Technology, an Asheville, North Carolina-based company, sells Play Attention. Peter Freer, a former science teacher and former technologist for the Asheville City Schools, founded the company in 1994.[6]

How it works:

Play Attention's method is to train a parent or other person to be a "coach" for the child as well as how to use the helmet and software. The initial training usually takes about three hours to learn but it is recommended that one use their support staff continuously to be sure that the system is properly employed. This is done via a distance learning program, which includes multimedia and communicating with one of their professionals on the phone or through e-mail. Program data are regularly uploaded and sent back to their support staff to provide continuous monitoring and evaluation of the child's progress.

This type of EEG biofeedback is performed utilizing three sensors that are fixed on the inside of a helmet. The helmet is placed on the individual's head to monitor the brainwaves. A saline solution is used to enhance the contact. The helmet is similar to one worn while biking.

The wires from the sensors pick up the brainwave frequencies and transfer them to the child's own personal computer loaded with special software to provide the EEG biofeedback. The frequencies that are rewarded and inhibited are fixed which simplifies the process.

One important area where Play Attention differs from traditional EEG biofeedback is that the focus is not on changing brainwave patterns but rather on producing cognitive changes that will in turn bring about an improvement in the behavior and performance of the child. To do this, Play Attention combines the use of EEG biofeedback with Edufeedback software to develop new cognitive skills. As a result, operant conditioning is integrated with cognitive skills training and behavior shaping.

The Play Attention® system covers five essential classroom skills. Each of these skills is described below:

> Level I is "Learning to Focus and Lessening Distractibility." The child begins his/her experience by working with a hierarchical series of games designed to increase the ability to attend for gradually increasing periods of time. By focusing on a fish swimming or a bird flying, the child can begin to understand that he/she can control the action on the screen merely by paying attention.
> Level II is "Visual Tracking." A child struggling with this skill may find it difficult to visually follow a teacher around the classroom. During this level, the child moves a character around the screen by focusing on it. The individual's scores are directly related to the time spent maintaining attention to the character's movements of the screen.
> Level III is "Time On-Task." At this level, the child practices building a tower of blocks, with the goal being to gradually decrease the time it takes to successfully build a tower. Accomplishing the task in less than five min-

utes is the objective. Blocks are carried across the screen by maintaining focus and are halted or moved backward if the child becomes off-task.

Level IV is "Short-Term Memory Sequencing." As implied by its name, this exercise focuses on increasing an individual's short-term memory, especially in increasingly longer sequences. The child concentrates on various colored blocks presented on the screen. The blocks light up in two, three, and four-light sequences. A unique tone is assigned to each block. After watching and hearing the sequence, the child must reproduce the sequence by inputting information with the keyboard.

Level V is "Discriminatory Processing." A cyber starship is the setting for this activity. As asteroids fly toward the ship, it is the child's task to deflect certain colored asteroids, but not others. In accomplishing this assignment, he or she is learning to pay attention to important stimuli while ignoring unimportant, irrelevant information.[7]

The coach and support staff continuously work with the child to ensure transfer and generalization of these skills. One way this is done is through a journal entry which the child completes after logging out of a session. In this journal entry, the child reflects on how these skills will be implemented at home or at school. During this same time period, it is the coach's job to set behavioral and cognitive objectives.

Play Attention says that this system improves focus, attention, visual tracking, time on task, short term memory, and discriminatory processing. Over time, the brain learns to produce these results without the aid of this system.

Sessions:

Training sessions usually last from 30 to 45 minutes. The sessions are usually conducted two times a week. At least 40 to 60 hours (not sessions) of training are suggested for long term benefits to occur. Therefore, parents might expect for their child to continue the training for at least 80 to100 sessions or 10 to12 months based on two times a week. It is also suggested that weaning the child off the program would be better than stopping the sessions all at once. This may add a little more time to the overall length of the program than what is stated above, but it may be well worth it. The reason that this process takes longer than other types of EEG biofeedback is that this system is designed to teach cognitive skills and shape behaviors, not train brainwaves.

Providers:

There are two main categories or types of providers. One is the professional who usually has a degree in a related field and has the capacity of training a number of children at one time. Examples of this are some educators who are using this system in schools. Other professionals such as mental health professionals may also use this system to provide this training for their clients. Yet another example is the "learning center," where this training is provided as part of an overall program to help kids with a variety of learning problems. A professional system is $2,495 with unlimited users.

The other type of provider is the individual, usually a parent of a child with ADHD, who gets the system for their family's own personal use. One of the advantages of this system is that interested parents may actually purchase it, and after a relatively short period of training, can become their own provider for their child under careful professional supervision.

Cost:

The cost of becoming a provider for one or two of your children is $1,795. This includes the training and the Play Attention® software, helmet, training, full support, and peripherals. It does not include the computer. However, the software will run on most home computers so if you already have your own computer, there should be no additional cost. Purchasing the system has an advantage in that there are no additional costs if you need to do more sessions than expected.

If you go to a professional that provides this training, the cost may vary greatly with sessions usually ranging from $25 to $65. When considering between 80 and 100 sessions, you could anticipate expenses ranging from $3,600 to $4,500. We have read, however, of at least one location on Long Island where the rate was $100 per session, so you find costs differing depending on your location.

Research:
Case Study in School Setting

Several case studies involving the use of Play Attention have been documented. In one of these studies, a second grade boy could solve math problems in his head, but could not successfully transfer this information to paper. His distractibility made it difficult for him to complete in-class tasks as well as homework assignments; he also displayed various impulsive behaviors in the classroom, including calling out inappropriately.

Within weeks of beginning sessions with a teacher who used Play Attention in the classroom and in private tutoring sessions, the boy began to control his impulsive actions and began to understand he had control over his own behaviors. At the end of the school year, this same child scored in the 99th percentile for math on the North Carolina end-of-year test.[8]

Case Studies in Clinical Setting

Two successful case studies in a clinical setting have also been reported.[9] Two boys, ages 6 ½ and 10, were assessed before and after their Play Attention training with a standardized test for measuring attention, called the Integrated Visual and Auditory Continuous Performance Test (IVA CPT). The IVA test scores are normalized identically to the more familiar IQ.

On the IVA's Response Control Quotient (RCQ), the younger boy scored 92 before and 99 after his training while the older child scored 81 before and 114 after training. A higher RCQ indicates lower impulsivity and faster reaction times.

In addition, the IVA produces an Attention Quotient (AQ) which corresponds to increased attention and attention stamina. The ability of both boys to pay attention and their attention stamina increased after the training. The 6 ½-year-old had a score of 64 before his training, and a score of 107 after the training. The 10-year-old's AQ score went from 103 to 121 after using Play Attention.

Additionally, other behaviors reported by the parents of these boys included fewer arguments at home, sitting and reading books with them, having normal social interactions, and being attentive in their classes at schools. Better social and academic reports were also received from their teachers.

Elementary School Study

A study conducted at Old Fort Elementary in Old Fort, North Carolina, examined the results of seven students with 20 or more hours of Play Attention training.[10] Six of the seven children increased their time on-task from 40% to 50% to nearly 100%. All seven students showed improvement in the areas of short-term memory sequencing and discriminatory processing. Also, their ability to sequence data increased from only two chunks to five or six chunks while the processing errors decreased from 20% to 0%.

According to its website, Play Attention is used throughout the world and in over 400 school systems in the United States. Although there are no large-scale scientific studies that prove the effectiveness of Play Attention, the State University of New York at Plattsburgh, East Virginia Medical School, and New Jersey schools under guidance from Duke University are currently studying the system with results expected by the end of 2005 or in early 2006.

Results:

Play Attention says that results can usually be seen in about four to six weeks if training is provided two times a week. Studies suggest that long-term benefits occur after 40 to 60 hours (not sessions) of training.

Pros & cons:

Cautions: This system is limited to those who only have difficulty with focus and attention. The Play Attention website reports no adverse side effects and equates the risk of using this product with using a telephone. However, Play Attention does recommend that individuals who experience anxiety or unpleasant feelings while using the system should not use it. They also say that it is not appropriate for children under six years of age and those who have an IQ below 65. Those who have other compounding issues such as seizures, closed head trauma, mental retardation, or fetal alcohol syndrome should consult a healthcare professional before using Play Attention.

Time: Although it takes a substantial number of hours to do the complete training, this program has the advantage of having maximum flexibility when choosing the day and time of doing the trainings, if you the parent are the provider.

Convenience: This is one of the primary benefits of this system. It can be done at home under the supervision of trained parents and does not require the services of a professional EEG biofeedback provider.

Recommended reading and websites:

www.playattention.com

Contact information:

Unique Logic and Technology, Inc.

1 Botany Drive, Suite 1F
Asheville, NC 28805-1607
Phone: 1-800-788-6786
E-mail: general@playattention.net

S.M.A.R.T. BrainGames

Names:

S.M.A.R.T. (Self Mastery and Regulation Training) BrainGames™
BrainGames
Smart Games

What it is:

This training is a combination of a home-based EEG neurofeedback system that can be combined with professional expertise. While a professional "Network Provider" sets up the overall program for a diagnosed condition, most of the actual training is done at the child's home. The system is completely compatible with off-the-shelf Sony PlayStation® video games. Unlike other EEG neurofeedback systems, the child uses hand-held game controls to play the game. It also does not require a computer except for analyzing the data to see how well the child is improving or if protocol changes are needed.

It uses technology developed by NASA scientists for the improvement of a pilot's attention and engagement to task. For years, scientists from NASA's Langley Research Center have been researching and developing various methods for assessing sustained attention, engagement, awareness, and pilot stress in laboratory flight simulators. One of the outgrowths of this biofeedback research is known as Extended Attention Span Training (EAST). EAST takes the form of a video game which responds to brain electrical activity and joystick input. CyberLearning Technology, LLC, the company that developed S.M.A.R.T. BrainGames and first released the system in 2003, is the only official NASA licensee for NASA's EAST Technologies.[11]

According to Alan Pope, a psychologist from NASA's Langley Research Center and co-inventor of EAST, violent video games are not recommended.

Car racing, skateboarding, and other skills-type games are best suited for this interactive technology.[12]

How it works:

A S.M.A.R.T. BrainGames "Network Provider" first evaluates the child. The child and his or her parents are then given their first session and taught how to set up and operate the system. Since it uses the standard Sony PlayStation video game system and does not require a computer, this training can usually be done in about one hour.

A helmet-like system, with electrodes embedded in it, is worn by the child to monitor the brainwaves and send them to the EEG neurofeedback device called the "Smart Box." A water-based electrolyte solution is used to improve the conductivity of the electrodes. The electrodes can be moved to a number of different sites on the head so that training can take place at different locations. This flexibility allows for several different training protocols to be used.

The child then simply plays an off-the-shelf video game using the modified S.M.A.R.T. Game Controller which looks very similar to the controller that comes with the PlayStation Game Platform. The primary difference is that the S.M.A.R.T. Game Controller communicates with the "Smart Box" via a wireless connection. The "Smart Box" receives the brainwaves from the helmet and analyzes them. Then, based upon the child's focus and attention, it allows the hand-held controls to become more or less effective.

For example, the system tracks the frequency of a child's brainwaves while playing a racing game in which the goal is to post a fast time to qualify for the next race. As a result, the player needs to maintain both speed and control. When the player exhibits low-frequency patterns, his race car slows and other cars pass him. That gets the player's attention so he concentrates, producing higher-frequency brainwaves. As a result his car gains speed, thereby providing positive reinforcement for his increased focus. The idea is that the higher-frequency pattern will continue for the child even after playing the game has stopped. In essence, according to CyberLearning Technology, the child's brain is the "accelerator" while the player's calmness is the "steering."

Sessions:

Training sessions usually last from 30 to 45 minutes and can be done daily or a few times a week. The overall length of the training varies with the need of the individual and can range from 50 to 100s of training sessions.

S.M.A.R.T. BrainGames allows for continued training even over the span of years since the motivating use of video games as the training display and the at-home convenience provides a unique and cost-effective training environment. Families can even view their ongoing training progress through sophisticated "SMART Software" designed to track progress and send training data to their "Network Provider" for remote viewing.

While the training program is in progress, periodic visits to the "Network Provider" will need to be made if the child has been diagnosed with a condition such as ADHD. The number and timing of these visits may vary, depending upon the need of the client. During these visits, the child's progress will be reviewed, the data from the system will be analyzed, and changes to the training protocol will be made as needed.

Providers:

The professional providers of this system are called "Network Providers." They are usually professionals in the medical or mental health fields who have received training in the use of EEG neurofeedback. Each provider has a geographic territory and can be found by looking on the S.M.A.R.T. BrainGames website (www.smartbraingames.com). These individuals are the only highly trained professionals able to provide this training for someone who has been diagnosed with a disorder such as ADHD.

Some people may want to use this system for non-clinical purposes such as peak performance training or just because it adds another dimension to playing video games. S.M.A.R.T. BrainGames has released an 'edutainment' version of the NASA based technology. For these people, this system can be purchased from the company by ordering directly through the on-line store at the company's website.

Cost:

The system costs $548. This cost is the same regardless if it is purchased from the Network Provider or directly from the company. Some Network Providers will sell you the system directly and some will ask that you buy it from the company and then they will provide the clinical supervision. In some cases, a Network Provider may lease out the system to an individual.

There are also professional expenses that the Network Provider will charge. These vary with the provider but usually range from $75 to $100 per visit. An additional expenditure will be the initial evaluation fee by the provider, which will probably cost more than $100. When adding up all of the costs, the charges of this training will likely total somewhere around $1,500.

On a negative side, you have to continue paying the monthly fee of $14.95 for a year under contract and continue paying the fee for as long as you keep the equipment. In order to stop the monthly fees, you have to return the equipment which you paid for in the beginning.

The PRO system can treat up to three people. This will reduce the cost per child for families with more than one family member who has ADHD.

Research:
Video Game Biofeedback vs. Traditional Neurofeedback

Researchers from NASA's Langley Research Center and the Eastern Virginia Medical School compared the differences between the use of video game biofeedback and traditional biofeedback with 22 children (19 boys and 3 girls) ranging in age from 9 to 13.[13] All of the participants had been diagnosed with ADHD of the hyperactive-impulsive subtype (DSM-IV) and were on short-acting medications for their ADHD.

The study assessed whether the videogame biofeedback technology developed at the Langley Research Center was as effective as traditional neurofeedback in treating ADHD and whether there were significant differences in its appeal. Eleven of the children received traditional biofeedback training while the other 11 played the modified video games. Participants were usually seen once or twice a week.

Following 40 one-hour training sessions, both groups showed significant improvements in everyday brainwave patterns as well as in tests measuring attention span, impulsiveness, and hyperactivity. Additionally, parents in both groups reported that their children were doing better in school.

Consequently, the researchers concluded that the video game biofeedback technology produced equivalent results to standard neurofeedback in effects on ADHD symptoms. Both the videogame and standard neurofeedback improved the functioning of all the children substantially above the benefits of medication alone.

It appeared, however, that there was a difference between the groups in the area of motivation. The video game group was more motivated, as evidenced by no drop-outs and fewer "no-shows" for testing. Parents of the video game group appeared to be more satisfied with the results of the training, and the children in that subgroup seemed to have more fun.

Parental Testimonial

As part of an article in *Business Week*, Dr. Elizabeth Ortiz-Natoli, a pediatrician who lives in Yorktown, Virginia, reported the benefits of S.M.A.R.T. BrainGames for her 11-year-old son.[14] She noted that her son was able to stop taking medications for his ADHD after taking part in a clinical study using this system developed by CyberLearning Technology. In this same article, it was acknowledged that more research is needed to establish just how useful the new generation of video games is in promoting better health. CyberLearning Technology stresses that its system should be viewed as an adjunct and complimentary training to medicine, not as a competitor.

Results:

S.M.A.R.T. BrainGames says that initial results should be seen in about 20 sessions. More significant results can be seen by about 35 sessions. However, this system has only recently been developed and so the results noted here include approximately a two-year time period. The company reports that they have not had to do any "booster" or follow up sessions during that time and that the benefits appear to be long standing.

Pros & cons

Cautions: Since the system has only been operating for approximately two years, the long-term results of this particular type of EEG neurofeedback are unknown.

Time: As with other EEG neurofeedback treatments, this one takes a substantial amount of time. With each session taking 45 minutes to one hour and being done six days a week for approximately 100 sessions, individuals have to be willing to adapt their daily schedules if they are going to use this method. Add in the time it takes to visit the provider several times and you can easily see that the time commitment can be great. This is especially true if there is not a provider in your immediate area.

Convenience: This can be viewed as both a pro and a con. Being able to do the training a home has its advantages, while having to travel to one of the Network Providers is a disadvantage. Since Network Providers are not located in all fifty states, finding a provider in your geographic area could present itself as a sizeable challenge.

Recommended reading and websites:

www.smartbraingames.com

Contact information:

CyberLearning Technology, LLC.
310 S. Twin Oaks Valley Road
Suite 107-296
San Marcos, CA 92078
Phone: (877) 860-6156
E-mail: info@smartbraingames.com

3

Interactive Metronome

Name:

Interactive Metronome® (IM)

What it is:

The Interactive Metronome (IM) was developed in the early 1990s. The treatment is based on the theory that the brain's motor planning and sequencing abilities influence a wide range of functions, including attention and concentration.[1]

Research has clearly shown that the brain learns through repetition of precise activities. Through the repetition of interactive exercises, IM strengthens the brain's ability to plan, sequence, and process information more effectively.

During IM exercises children wear headphones and listen to a rhythmic computer-generated metronome beat. At the sound of each beat, the children attempt to perform a prescribed movement, such as hand clapping or foot tapping. Sensors measure how accurately the children are able to perform the exercise in conjunction with the beat. Later in the exercises the IM generates another set of sounds and visual cues that provide the children immediate feedback on how closely they are matching the beat. Those guide sounds and visual cues cause the children to concentrate further and to use the sounds and screen to improve their performance on the IM. The IM progressively challenges children to improve their score. In doing so they are exercising attention, sensory integration, and neuro-motor synchronization.

According to the IM website (www.interactivemetronome.com), the IM has been used for years with children diagnosed with ADD/ADHD, in addition to Sensory Integration Disorder, Asperger's, Autism Spectrum Disorder, and Cerebral Palsy. However, Dr. Stanley I. Greenspan, chairman of the Interactive Metronome, Inc. Scientific Advisory Committee, as well as a nationally recognized child psychiatrist and author, clarifies that IM is not targeted for any specific syndrome, but rather improves motor planning and sequencing skills for many children. He acknowledges that IM helps with ADHD, but that IM can also be helpful for any attention problems, distractibility, and poor motor coordination. Children without any special conditions or problems may also find it beneficial.[2]

How it works:

In addition to the Interactive Metronome software program, the IM package includes two sets of headphones and two contact sensing triggers. One trigger, a special glove with a contact sensor attached to the palm side, senses exactly when the triggered hand makes contact with the other hand while clapping, or when one hand is tapped on the thigh. The other trigger, a flat pad placed on the floor, senses when a toe or heel is tapped upon it. When an individual taps a limb in time with the steady metronome reference beat, the trigger sends a signal to the IM computer program.[3] The resulting distance between the IM generated beat and the child's actual hand or foot strike is measured in milliseconds and is the basis for the child's IM score. A low millisecond score indicates improved timing and overall performance. Thus, the lower the IM score, the more progress is occurring.

During IM's eleven years of research they have determined the normative range scores according to age. Therefore after each exercise, participants are shown their scores on the computer screen and are encouraged by their progress. Receiving immediate feedback appears to serve as a positive motivational technique. Pre, mid and post-tests are administered during IM treatment, which allow the IM trainer to monitor progress.

Each IM session includes a given number of thirteen hand and foot exercises that are repeated a specific number of times as prescribed in the daily treatment routine guide. However, the exercises may be modified to meet each child's individual needs.

There is also an assessment component of IM which takes approximately 20 minutes to complete and is used to evaluate whether an individual would benefit from the IM program treatment. Many IM providers offer this session free of charge or for a reduced fee.

Sessions:

Typically, the duration of treatment is 12 to 15 sessions. Three to five treatment sessions per week are suggested. Therefore, the treatment can be completed in three to five weeks. However, as with any treatment, the number of sessions will depend upon the individuals and their response to this treatment.

Providers:

According to the IM website, those qualified for certification include individuals who are licensed, degreed, or certified in healthcare or developmental rehabilitation services, special education, and other related disciplines. Such professionals include occupational therapists, physical therapists, speech/language pathologists, audiologists, psychologists, educators, psychiatrists, and pediatricians.[4]

Interactive Metronome certifies those individuals who are eligible to become IM providers. A link on the IM official website (www. interactivemetronome.com) provides a listing of IM providers by zip code, by city, or by state.

Cost:

IM does not regulate or recommend the cost charged by their providers. Some IM providers charge per session and some charge for a set of sessions. The cost varies depending upon who is providing the treatment. Most providers charge a comparable amount to what their profession usually charges. Information gathered shows a cost per session from $65 to $125. As a result, the total cost for 15 sessions would range from $975 to $1,875.

Generally speaking, insurance does not cover ADHD and would therefore not reimburse for IM treatment provided for those diagnoses. In cases where the diagnosis is covered by insurance IM can be billed under general therapy codes for reimbursement purposes. To find a definite answer, your specific coverage questions will need to be addressed to your insurance company.

Research:
Timing and Rhythmicity: Their Impact on Academic Performance Study

One study involving 316 boys and 269 girls found significant correlations between Interactive Metronome timing and academic performance in reading, math, language, science, social studies, and study skills.[5] The 585 participants were between the ages of 4 and 11. Results indicate that timing and rhythmicity (any type of activity requiring that children coordinate sound and vibration with movement) play a foundational role in the cognitive processes underlying performance in these academic areas. A strong relationship between attentiveness in class and better timing and rhythmicity was also found.

Matched Groups: Interactive Metronome vs. Video Games vs. Control

Fifty-six boys diagnosed with ADHD, ranging in age from 6 to 12, were pre-tested and assigned to one of three matched groups. This study was conducted over a three-week period The subgroup receiving 15 hours of IM treatment was compared with a group receiving no treatment and another group receiving therapy on selected video games. Children receiving IM treatment improved in the areas of attention, motor control, language processing, and reading.[6] In addition, parents reported improvement in their child's control of aggressive behavior after the IM treatment.

Discussion

Although the matched groups study was a carefully conducted research study, it is essential to recognize some of its limitations. Since this study was limited to boys, the potential benefit of this treatment for girls with ADHD is uncertain. Because all participants were already receiving medication, the value of IM treatment for ADHD in the absence of medication is unclear. It is important to recognize, however, that because the boys were apparently already benefiting from their medication treatment, the fact that the Interactive Metronome treatment resulted in additional gains is certainly encouraging.

Another limitation is that no additional follow-up was conducted. Therefore, it is still unknown whether the benefits of IM treatment would be sustained over time. A final concern is that the specific pre- and post-treatment scores were not included with the results, so the actual magnitude of the gains resulting from the Interactive Metronome treatment could not be examined.[7]

This specific research study is discussed in the September 2002 issue of *Attention Research Update.* The results of this study seem to indicate that IM treatment may play a useful role in the treatment of ADHD. However, additional research studies addressing this study's limitations were called for in order to determine the usefulness of IM treatment as an adjunctive or possibly even a primary treatment for ADHD.[8]

The same promising view of IM treatment is echoed in the CHADD Fact Sheet #6, entitled "Assessing Complementary and Controversial Interventions." It does caution, however, that more research is necessary before the value of IM can be known with greater certainty.[9]

IM reports that several studies are currently underway or in development with independent agencies. One multi-site large-scale ADHD study is investigating how a broad spectrum of outcomes resulting from treatment with a combination of IM and medication compare with those from medication alone.

Another study being conducted at a large public high school is quantifying the effects of Interactive Metronome treatment on academic performance on a wide range of measures by means of standardized test scores. An elementary academic performance study involving third and fourth graders is examining IM's impact on proficiency in reading and math and working memory.

IM is currently used in over 100 rehabilitation hospitals to help treat adult patients with Parkinson's disease, strokes or traumatic brain injuries. It is also used by a number of university and professional teams to improve sports performance.[10]

In recommending the IM to parents, one provider, an occupational therapist in North Carolina, recommended doing the sessions after school, on weekends, and during the summer and/or early fall. In this way the children would be able to see their progress clearly throughout the school year.[11]

Results:

According to the IM website, case studies monitored over the past ten years illustrate that lasting effects may be obtained after completing the IM program. Patients tested six and 12 months post-treatment demonstrate almost identical performance on the IM as accomplished during the treatment process.

Pros & cons:

Cautions: An eligible candidate for IM needs to be at the developmental age of six years or older. The one major research study dealing with ADHD only dealt with boys who were already on medication, so the value of IM treatment for ADHD in the absence of medication is uncertain. There is no published research on its benefit for girls with ADHD.

Time: There are a set number of sessions. The program typically involves 12 to 15 sessions with sessions recommended at least two times per week. The entire program could be completed in a four to five-week timeframe.

Convenience: Since all providers must complete Interactive Metronome certification, you will need to find a provider practicing in your geographic area. There are currently over 3,000 certified IM providers in the United States. They can be located using the "Locate an IM Provider" option at www.interactivemetronome.com.

Other: IM is a non-invasive procedure with no documented adverse effects.

Recommended reading and websites:

Shaffer, R.J., Jacokes, L.E., Cassily, J.F., Greenspan, S.I., Tuchman, R.F., & Stemmer, P.J. (2001). Effect of interactive metronome treatment on children with AD/HD. *The American Journal of Occupational Therapy, 55,* 155-162.

www.interactivemetronome.com
www.chadd.org/fs/fs6.htm
www.helpforadd.com/2002/september.htm
www.highscope.org/Research/TimingPaper/timingstudy.htm
www.specialkidstoday.com/resources

Contact information:

2500 Weston Road, Suite 403
Weston, Florida 33331
Toll Free: (877) 994-6776

Phone: (954) 385-4660
Fax: (954) 385-4674
E-mail: info@interactivemetronome.com

4

Light and Sound Therapies

* Audio-Visual Entrainment (AVE) Devices

* Binaural Beats

Light and sound therapies use flashing lights and/or sounds in order to impact the brain's functioning through a phenomenon known as "entrainment." Here, brainwaves match and resonate at the same frequency as the stimulating light and/or sound. For example, if you have two tuning forks of the same pitch, if one is struck and held near the other, they will both resonate at the same frequency. It also works with two pianos. If you have two similarly tuned pianos in a room and strike a key on one piano, the stretched chord attached to the same key on the other piano will vibrate. This principle of entrainment can be used to resonate, synchronize, or tune the brain to specific frequencies. Entrainment is also used to reduce the slow brainwave activity that is abnormally high in children with ADHD.

The process of reproducing this "entrainment effect" using audio technology was discovered in 1934 by Adrian and Matthews and further developed in the 1950s. Rhythmic sound waves entering the ears result in a portion of the brainwave frequency resonating to the stimulating audio frequency. While some sound waves can cause the brainwaves to slow down and relax thereby reducing anxiety, other more stimulating frequencies can perk up brain functioning and help the brain to perform better.

Entrainment to visual stimulation occurs when rhythmic lights flashed into an individual's eyes cause the brainwave pattern of the cortex to fall into the same frequency as the flashing or flickering light. Both light and sound therapies work in much the same way in that they both use sensory input to influence the functioning of the brain.

The technology of light and sound therapies is not as simple as it may first appear. Although you may feel calmer after listening to relaxing music, simply listening to a stimulating song will not help your brain to function better. What must occur to help with ADHD is for the right frequencies to be utilized in the right way under the right conditions for a particular desired effect. In researching this technology we found two modalities, with some research studies, that appear to be effective in helping to treat ADHD. They are Audio-Visual Entrainment (AVE) and binaural beats.

Audio-Visual Entrainment (AVE) Devices

Names:

Light and Sound Machines
Mind Machines
Audio-Visual Entrainment/AVE
Audio-Visual Stimulation/AVS
The "DAVID" (Digital Audio-Visual Integration Device)

What it is:

Audio-Visual Entrainment (AVE) devices use both flashes of lights and pulses of tones to affect the brainwave frequencies. There are several companies that sell these products and each product is somewhat different in its features.

Since it is not within the scope of this book to list every product and explain its particular characteristics, we will only discuss one of the leading products in this area. By doing so, you should gain a basic understanding of all AVE devices. The information we will be covering is on the "DAVID," a product developed by Mind Alive Inc. We selected this product as it is one with which we are familiar, having used it personally and professionally.

How it works:

The equipment consists of headphones, eyesets, and a small box, which is the generating device. Lights flash at predetermined frequencies through the pair of eyesets. These eyesets are made from a pair of oversized sunglasses with tiny lights on the inside. Sound takes the form of pulsating tones delivered through the pair of headphones. Either the headphones and eyesets can pulse at the same frequencies or they can generate different frequencies on the left and right sides. This enables training to take place where the whole brain can be synchronized or the left and right brain can be entrained at different frequencies.

Rather than these pulsations being annoying, the light and sound frequencies actually provide a focus for the mind, quieting the mental chatter and making it easy for the individual to relax and enjoy the session. After a short period of time, the brainwave frequencies will resonate or entrain to the same frequencies as the light and sound stimulus. Depending upon the protocol chosen the brain can be entrained to become more activated, less activated, or simply exercised. In this way, it is similar to EEG neurofeedback except here the brain is driven to a different level of functioning rather than rewarded for going there on its own.

While parents might want to use this therapy to reduce anxiety by slowing their brainwaves down, the child with ADHD will need speedier brainwaves to treat his/her slow brainwave disorder. As you may surmise, this is similar to the effect that stimulant medication has on the brain. After a number of sessions, the brain learns how to start producing more of these desired frequencies on its own.

In addition to the effect that the light and sound frequencies have on the brain, there are also additional features which guide the individual with breath pacing and/or heart rate regulation. Tapes or CDs can also be easily connected to the system to add another dimension to the entrainment and to make the training more interesting for the child.

Sessions:

Various training sessions are programmed into the system so that you only have to select the pre-programmed session number, which fits the specific issue that you wish to target. In this case, you will be selecting a session specifically designed for ADHD. Once the eyesets and headphones are placed on the head and a session has been selected, the device runs a sequence of frequencies automatically and shuts off when the sequence is completed.

The time of the session is pre-programmed from the factory. However, software may be purchased to allow the user to custom program the "DAVID" system as desired. Most of the sessions dealing with ADHD range from about 20 to 30 minutes and are usually done on a daily basis. Since most of the gains will be made in about the first 40 sessions, after that time the child may be reduced to just one session a week or none at all. However, there are some children who may need to continue frequent use in order to maintain their improvements.

Since AVE is very flexible, it can also be used on a variety of conditions associated with ADHD. If your child has a lot of anxiety, the sessions usually start with a relaxing program, which helps the child learn to relax and become more stable. If falling asleep is an issue, there are programs that will help with bringing about the onset of sleep. After a week or two, the relaxing programs are replaced with sessions done in the morning that are higher in frequency and are meant to stimulate the brain and increase its functioning, much the same as a stimulant medication. These sessions can be "played" while children are still in bed before they start their day.

Providers:

Parents can purchase the equipment and use the system with very little training. There are some mental health and educational professionals who use this product as part of their professional practice. For simple ADHD issues, most parents can be effective in utilizing this system without the use of a professional provider. However, for more complex issues, finding a professional provider is recommended.

Cost:

The primary cost is the equipment. Prices range from approximately $100 to $650. Since you are getting this equipment for clinical purposes, you might want to stay away from the lesser expensive models. By purchasing a system in the middle price range, you will probably get better technology, which should produce better results.

Insurance will generally not cover the cost of this equipment, as it is not a medical device. However, the cost of this equipment is relatively inexpensive when compared to other therapies discussed in this book.

Research:
Pilot Study of AVE with Learning Disabled Boys

This study focused on the effects of auditory and visual stimulation (AVS) training on the academic and behavioral functioning of 26 learning disabled boys, who attended either a private or public school.[1] All of the boys were between the ages of 8 and 12.

Each participant was administered a group of pre- and posttests which included the following: Peabody Picture Vocabulary Test (to measure verbal IQ), Raven Coloured Progressive Matrices (to measure non-verbal IQ), Auditory Sequential Memory subtest of the Illinois Test of Psycholinguistic Abilities, Wechsler Intelligence Scale for Children-Revised, Wide Range Achievement Test-Revised (for reading, spelling, and math), Burks' Behavior Rating Scale (completed by teachers and parents). All testing was conducted during the week prior to the AVS treatment and during the week following the last AVS treatment.

Each of the 14 participants attending the private school received a total of 40 AVS treatments, given in a group setting to four or five students at a time. The sessions were administered in a designated room at school five days a week for eight weeks. The AVS was preset to operate for a total of 25 minutes in a cycle that was repeated five times. In addition, the boys were asked to use a special relaxation tape at home for five days a week for eight weeks. The tape had the same pattern of sound stimulation used in the AVS at school.

In contrast, the 12 participants who attended public school only received three treatments weekly for six weeks, totaling 18 treatments in all. Not surprisingly, the results of the group receiving the 40 therapy sessions were considerably better.

Significant differences were found on four of the six assessment measures for the children receiving more sessions. Statistically significant improvements were noted in non-verbal IQ scores, memory, reading scores, and spelling scores, as well as on the behavioral rating scale. Only the changes in the Peabody Picture Vocabulary Test and the math score on the Wide Range Achievement Test did not show significant improvement.

According to the boys' teachers, every scale score on the Burks' Behavior Rating Scale was lower at the posttest than at the pretest. In general, lower scores indicate improvement on this behavioral measure. Parents' ratings showed the children's scores lower on 17 of the 19 possible scales. Both teachers and parents rated the "poor attention" and the "poor academics" scales as significantly improved.

Discussion

According to Carter and Russell, the researchers who conducted this pilot study, the results indicate that AVS training may be a simpler and lower-cost alternative to EEG training. They view this procedure as less threatening and demanding on the students being trained than the EEG training model where the child is required to learn how to recognize and produce the desired brainwaves in amplitude and/or frequency. The training time required for the child to learn to recognize and bring about improved concentration or attention appears to be accomplished in a relatively short period of time. Finally, the researchers suggest that the simplicity of using the AVS and the low cost of the equipment may make effective treatment available to many children who need it but who would perhaps otherwise never receive it.

AVE as Treatment for Behavior Disorders in School Setting

Thirty-four elementary children (21 boys, 13 girls) from two different schools were given AVE treatment over a seven-week period.[2] A majority of the students had a history of distractibility and misbehavior. In addition, 14 of the children had either been diagnosed as ADHD or were suspected to be ADHD while 10 were reported as having an unspecified learning disorder.

Participants, ranging in age from 8 to 11, were administered the Test of Variables of Attention (TOVA) before and after the treatment period. The TOVA is a continuous performance assessment used to measure inattention, impulsivity, reaction time, and variability.

In addition, eight of the participants were also in a special reading class and were evaluated on the Standardized Test for the Assessment of Reading (STAR) as well as the TOVA. The STAR is a computed-based, norm-referenced reading test.

The AVE treatment sessions were given Monday-Friday for seven weeks beginning early in the fall semester. The AVE device used in the study was the DAVID Paradise XL, which is manufactured by Comptronic Devices Limited.

A total of 35 sessions were provided, with students receiving from 28 to 33 sessions. Sessions took place in a quiet, dimly lit room at each school site. The first eight sessions were 20 minutes in length; the rest of the sessions were 22 minutes long.

Soon after the treatment sessions began, auditory stimulus was added to engage some of the children. Tapes used included environmental sounds, such as birds, insects, and rain, as well as instrumental music, such as strings and percussion. An individual tape was selected randomly for each session. All participants received stimulation from the selected tapes.

Results for the total group on the TOVA posttest showed improvement in all four TOVA areas. This improvement was statistically significant on the following three subscales: inattention, impulsivity, and variability. The eight students from the STAR program who also received AVE improved their reading scores more than their classmates who served as controls. Although no specific assessment instrument was used to measure improvements in student behavior, teachers and parents reported the children receiving the training were calmer and were better able to focus.

In the discussion section of their article, Siever and Joyce identified several reasons why AVE technology should be available in school settings. Among the explanations were the following: (1) most parents or communities that need technologies like AVE or neurofeedback the most can least afford it, (2) travel time is minimized or eliminated as a factor, (3) immediate and ongoing feedback and random on-site observations can more easily occur, and (4) medication dosages can be reduced. Finally, the researchers concluded that even though AVE appears cost-effective when comparing it to neurofeedback, it should not be viewed as capable of solving all behavioral or learning issues in a school setting.

Use of Auditory and Visual Stimulation to Treat ADHD

This doctoral dissertation study evaluated the effectiveness of stimulant medication treatment for ADHD (Ritalin and Adderall) and the effectiveness of a combination of medication and audio-visual stimulation (AVS) treatment options.[3] Ninety-nine children who had all been diagnosed with ADHD participated. The following four treatment groups were compared: (1) AVS group, (2) stimulant medication group, (3) AVS/stimulant medication group, and (4) self-selected comparison group.

The children participated in 20-minute treatment sessions five days a week for a total of 40 sessions. Although the researcher administered the first training session, the remaining 39 sessions were completed at home under the supervision of a parent or guardian.

Various assessments were used to determine the effectiveness of the four treatment options. The Wide Range Achievement Test—Revised, the Peabody Picture Vocabulary Test, and the Raven Progressive Matrices were used to measure cognitive functioning levels before and after treatment. The Attention Deficit Disorder Evaluation Scale and the Integrated Visual and Auditory Continuous Performance Test were used to assess behavioral changes. Testing was done just prior to the treatment, immediately following the last treatment session, and again four weeks following the completion of the treatment sessions.

Results indicated that both the AVS group and the combination AVS/ stimulant medication group showed significant statistical improvements in both cognitive and behavioral functions. In contrast, the group using stimulant medication alone demonstrated less improvement when compared to the AVS and combination of AVS/stimulant treatment groups. The self-selected control group showed no change on either cognitive or behavioral measures.

Michelletti, the doctoral student conducting this research study, was a social worker. In his concluding remarks the researcher commented that AVS is both relatively inexpensive and relatively easy to operate. While he reminded the reader that AVS treatment is not a "cure-all" for those diagnosed with ADHD, he did suggest that it could be an important adjunctive treatment option.

Neurotechnology Project Report

This study by Joyce involved seven public schools (five elementary, one middle, and one K-12) in Minnesota investigating the effects of using AVE to address inattention, impulsiveness, and behavioral challenges in a school-age population.[4] Children selected to participate had a history of learning and reading challenges, impulsiveness, and a tendency to be easily distracted and to distract others.

The DAVID Paradise XL, manufactured by Mind Alive Inc., was the AVE device used in this school project. Students received two or three 20 to 30-minute AVE sessions per week, for a period of 12 weeks. Participants averaged approximately 30 sessions during the treatment period.

Each child was assessed before and after the treatment period using the Slosson-R reading test. In addition, parents and teachers completed a behavior rating scale on each child.

Participants averaged an eight-month gain in their oral reading scores. Post-test scores on the behavior rating scales indicated a reduction in anxiety, depression, hyperactivity, and inattention.

Results:

If you use the system on a daily basis, you should begin to notice results within a week or two. For the next several months, the child should continue making steady improvements. After that time, the improvements may begin to taper off.

Pros & cons:

Cautions: This device is not recommended for individuals who are epileptic or get seizures from flashing lights (photo epileptic). It is recommended that anyone who has a history of brain seizures, mental disorders, or alcohol and/or drug abuse use this equipment only under the supervision of a medical doctor. Also, if a person has had any past traumatic experiences, suppressed memories may possibly be released as well.

Time: The time commitment for the sessions is minimal. Although the sessions are usually done on a daily basis, they are usually between 20-30 minutes and the equipment can be set up in only a few seconds.

Cost: The cost is relatively inexpensive as there is only the one time cost for the equipment. If you obtain services from a provider who uses this as part of therapy, then the cost may be substantially higher.

Convenience: This is one of the most convenient treatments for ADHD since it can be done at home and easily worked into your schedule. Also, with the exception of very young children, children can be taught to use the system by themselves. By getting the portable model, it can easily be carried around and used almost anywhere.

Other: One of the better features of this product is that training sessions are not limited to your child. As you already know, ADHD can be very stressing for parents as well. This additional stress can cause a variety of problems within the family such as anxiety, depression, and insomnia. A parent's stress level is often transferred to the child making him/her more stressed, which in turn, increases the child's inattentiveness, impulsiveness, and/or hyperactivity. When your child is not using the system, you can use the preset programs for a variety of issues of your own. As you are able to deal better with life's stressors, you may find that your child is able to calm down more easily as well.

Recommended reading and websites:

The Rediscovery of Audio-Visual Entrainment Technology
Author: Dave Siever
Mind Alive Inc. Copyright 2002

New Technology for Attention and Learning
Author: Dave Siever
Mind Alive Inc. Copyright 2003

www.mindalive.com
www.dynamind.com/ls.htm
www.toolsforwellness.com/light-sound-machines.html

Contact information:

Various types of light and sound machines can be obtained from the websites listed above. Since there are several companies that produce the different systems, we have chosen not to include all of them. However, for your convenience, we are listing the contact information on the company whose system we discussed in this chapter and specifically identified in two of the research studies.

Mind Alive, Inc.
9008-51 Avenue
Edmonton, Alberta, Canada
T6E 5X4
Phone: (800) 661-6463 (toll free Canada and U.S. only) (780) 450-3729
E-mail: info@mindalive.com

Binaural Beats

Names

Binaural Beats
Binaural Auditory Beats
Auditory Binaural Beat Stimulation

What it is:

When two tones of different frequencies are presented separately to each ear, the brain is able to synthesize the two sounds into a single low-frequency tone, which is the binaural beat. So, for example, if you have a beat frequency of 94 Hz in your left ear and 100 Hz in your right ear, your brain will perceive it as a 6 Hz differential. Your brain, therefore, will resonate at this 6 Hz frequency. In other words, a binaural beat of 6 Hz will be produced.

How it works:

Devices designed to create binaural beats send different sounds or tones to each ear through stereo headphones or properly placed stereo speakers. Acting in unison, the two hemispheres of the brain are then able to "hear" a third signal, which is the difference between the two tones. It is really not an actual sound, however, but rather an electrical signal which can only be perceived within the brain by both hemispheres working together.

If the difference between tones matches a particular brainwave state, such as the 4 to 8 Hz theta range, the 8 to 12 Hz alpha range, or the 12 to 24 Hz beta range, the overall brain activity will maintain that particular brainwave state. The brain will then begin to function at this level of arousal. Therefore, you can create the possibility of attaining a particular state of consciousness by varying the frequencies of the tones delivered to each ear, as well as by varying the differences between the two frequencies.

It is important to keep in mind, however, that delivering the appropriate frequencies to the listener's ears is only one factor in attaining a particular state of consciousness. The listener must also be cooperative and receptive in order for the signals to work. This is not an automatic process. A person can reject the effect if he or she so chooses.

Sessions:

There is no specific number of sessions recommended in treating ADHD. Since the research on binaural beats gives no indication of any positive carry-over beyond an hour or so after listening to the tapes, you might want to determine the occasions or circumstances when your child would benefit the most. Some of these times might be during homework, while riding to school, or during any situation when he or she needs to calm down.

Providers:

Although there are some professional providers or mental health professionals who may be using binaural beat recordings as an adjunct to other therapies they may offer, there are no official providers as such. Any individual can buy the items necessary to implement this modality for personal use. Binaural beat CDs, tapes, and equipment can be obtained directly from the companies listed in the contact section at the end of this chapter.

Cost:

Insurance will not cover the expense of this treatment option. However, since no providers are utilized, the cost to use this modality is minimal. The only expenditures would be a standard cassette or CD player and the binaural tapes or CDs. Most people already own the standard cassette or CD player needed. The cost for a binaural beat CD or tape will probably range from $20 to $40.

Research:
Using Binaural-Beat Stimulation with ADHD Children and Adults

This study, involving 11 individuals ranging in age from 6 to 43, tested whether auditory binaural-beat stimulation would result in an increase of beta brainwave activity in participants diagnosed with ADHD.[5] All participants were taking medication for their condition. Additionally, none of the individuals had any hearing impairment, past closed-head injury, or seizure disorder. The group was comprised of seven males (3 boys) and four females (1 girl).

The Monroe Institute specially produced two compact discs (CDs), both entitled *Einstein's Dream*, for this research project. The CD for the experimental phase of the study contained binaural-beat stimulation while the control-phase CD did not. To the ear the two CDs sounded identical. Battery-operated stereo headphones were used to listen to the CDs.

A modified version of the Conners' Continuous Performance Test (CPT) was used during each of the five "music" phases to measure participants' attentiveness scores. The five "music" phases were as follows: (1) two-minute baseline recording, (2) two-minute non-binaural beat recording, (3) four minutes of CPT while still listening to non-binaural beat music, (4) two-minute binaural-beat recording, and (5) four minutes of CPT while still listening to binaural-beat music.

Scores on the CPT were calculated during each of the five phases. In comparing the attentiveness scores during Phase II (non-binaural music) and Phase IV (binaural music), participants displayed a significantly higher attentiveness level during the binaural-beat recording phase. In addition, the results showed a significant increase in CPT attentiveness scores for the final or fifth phase.

According to the researcher, this finding gives additional support to the positive effect of the binaural-beat recording. He reports that Conners, the developer of the CPT, has indicated children normally become bored with the repetitive type of task measured by this assessment instrument. Therefore, a child's performance would likely decline the longer he or she is engaged in the task. Consequently it could be anticipated that the score in the final or fifth phase of the experiment might be lower. However, it is significant that this study's results do not follow that expected tendency. Instead, it appears that the positive effects of binaural beats last up to an hour or longer.

Using Binaural Beats to Enhance Attention with ADHD Children

The purpose of this study was to determine which specific patterns of sound, and which corresponding brainwave states, would be most effective in helping children diagnosed with ADHD feel alert or sustain attention.[6] Three different patterns or combinations of sound frequencies were used. Although 18 children, ranging in age from 6 to 14 years old, began as participants, only 11 children completed the study. The researcher had told the parents that if any resistance to listening occurred, they were not to force their child and simply to discontinue participating.

The children, who were all volunteered by their parents, were asked to listen to three different tapes using headphones. Each participant was given three tapes which had been randomly labeled either Tape A, Tape B, or Tape C. This procedure was done to reduce the influence of expectation and possible order effects on the outcome. The tapes had three variations of Hemi-Sync® tones embedded behind a musical score entitled *Heart Zones.*

Tape A was to be used for a one-week period with the child listening three or more times during the week. Next, Tape B was to be used for a one-week period with listening occurring three or more times. The third or final week, Tape C was to be listened to for three or more times.

The effectiveness of each tape was assessed through parent observation and feedback. Parents were asked to observe any changes in their child while the child was listening to a tape and/or engaged in an activity. They were asked to do an overall evaluation of which tape the child preferred most, as well as which tape best helped their child to stay focused. For each week, the parents were to document how many times the particular tape was used, any important observations, and whether the use of the tape corresponded with any specific changes in their child's eating or sleeping habits. They were also asked to record whether the child liked to use the tape and any other pertinent information they felt was important, including any changes in behavior at school.

Results of the study indicated that 8 of the 11 children preferred the tape with tones reinforcing brainwave activity at the 12 and 16 Hz level. The parents provided various informative and positive comments. Here are a few of the observations from the parents shared by the researcher:

- "If he listens to it before school, he's calmer and much easier to get along with."

- "Calmed him down. Attitude changed. Was pleasant to be around. (maybe because he slept better)."

- "…only a few minutes of this tape works wonders."

- "It was a positive experience for him and seemed to have a positive effect. Matt is very impulsive and explosive and that seemed to improve."

Two of the students who had no preference both reported better attention during an activity, although their parents reported no significant improvement.

There was a very strong preference for the tape with tones reinforcing 12 and 16 Hz brainwave activity. No participants preferred the 8 and 12 Hz combination. The researcher's observation was that this level is apparently too slow to provide the arousal necessary for ADHD children to sustain comfortable attention.

Results:

The results of these two studies support using binaural beat recordings to improve attentiveness and promote calming. It should be noted that during the first study, all of the participants were on medication. Therefore, we do not know if the positive results obtained would be reproduced without medication. Also, the studies do not show these effects to be long lasting. It appears that the positive effects of binaural beats may primarily be during the time of the listening and shortly thereafter.

Pros & cons:

Cautions: There appear to be no negative side effects and no limitations as to the age, mental, or physical conditions of those using binaural beats.

Time: The time commitment is minimal as there is no recommended number of times your child needs to use the tapes and no duration of time which the tapes need to be played when utilized.

Convenience: One of the strengths of using binaural beat tapes is the convenience. You can play the tapes almost anywhere and anytime. You also only need to use them during those times when your child needs to focus better such as when doing homework.

Recommended reading and websites:

www.monroeinstitute.org/research/hemisync/binaural.html
www.binaural-beats.com/binaural-beats.com
web-us.com/thescience.htm
uazu.net/sbagen
www.healthynewage.com/thepath.html
www.hemi-sync.com/shop/customer/home.php

Contact information:

Binaural beats products can be bought from several of the websites listed above. You may also find them at your local bookstore or music store.

5

Chiropractic

Names:

Chiropractic
Chiropractic Manipulation
Spinal Adjustment

What it is:

While chiropractic has been practiced for over 100 years in our country, its basic wellness practices date back to the first use of spinal manipulations by Hippocrates in the 4th Century B.C. The primary focus of chiropractic is the detection, reduction, and correction of spinal misalignments and nervous system dysfunction. Chiropractors are specialists in neuromusculoskeletal conditions.

Doctors of Chiropractic try to determine the cause of a health problem, rather than merely treating the symptoms. They attempt to maximize the natural strengths of the human body and its ability to heal itself. Chiropractors do not include medication or surgery in their treatment program, although nutritional, postural, and lifestyle modifications/recommendations are often part of chiropractic care.

How it works:

The expertise of the Doctor of Chiropractic lies in evaluating an individual's spine for misalignments that impair nervous system function, which impacts overall body function. The vertebrae house and protect the spinal cord. The spinal cord is an extension of the brain and carries information from the brain to the various parts of the body and back to the brain again. Subluxations, or misaligned vertebrae, interfere with the nervous system's ability to transmit this important information.

Through a series of adjustments, the Doctor of Chiropractic helps to restore the misaligned vertebrae to a more normal position, thereby allowing the nerves to communicate appropriately with the rest of the body. This, in turn, allows the body to heal itself naturally, without drugs or surgery.

Chiropractic adjustments by themselves do not heal the body. When any of the spinal vertebrae become misaligned, a basic imbalance or disruption can occur in the nervous and blood vascular systems. Such an imbalance or disruption may contribute to stress in the body.

The Doctor of Chiropractic will take a case history and perform a chiropractic exam to determine if spinal subluxations exist. Adjustment procedures are modified to fit a person's size, weight, and individual spinal condition.

Chiropractors use their hands in applying corrective pressure to the patient's spine in a specific direction and location. This procedure is known as "spinal adjustment." In some cases, they may use instrumentation to detect the slight dislocation or misalignment.

Misaligned vertebrae, known as subluxations, can irritate nerves and interfere with the body's ability to transmit messages through the spine to different parts of the body. All parts of the body need proper nerve energy and a flow of information in order to function properly. If the misalignment is not corrected, the spinal malfunction can cause pain, muscle and organ dysfunction, and other imbalances.

There are numerous causative factors for spinal misalignments in children. These factors include: traumatic birth, improper support of the neck during infancy, sleeping in car seats with the neck unsupported, standing/walking too early (which affects the proper development of the cervical curve), accidents or falls, repetitive strain while studying/watching television/playing video games, awkward sleeping positions, poor posture, and carrying heavy backpacks.

Since a subluxation can result from relatively simple causes and not just from a traumatic event, such as a car accident, you as the parent will probably not know if this is a factor in your child's ADHD-type behaviors. Many spinal misalignments do not cause pain or outward symptoms and can only be detected by a thorough examination by a Doctor of Chiropractic.

Some outward signs, however, may be observed by parents. These signs include: a tilted or rotated head or neck, a high shoulder or hip, difficulty turning the neck, neck stiffness or soreness to the touch, and rubbing of the neck, back of head, or ear. In older children, complaints of soreness, headaches, stiffness, or difficulty sleeping due to discomfort could occur.

In the case of ADHD, the problem is usually a subluxation in the upper cervical area of the neck. The C-1 vertebra, also known as the atlas, is a small donut-like bone located at the top of the spine and the base of the skull. The atlas surrounds the brain stem. A misalignment of the atlas vertebra affects the alignment of the entire spine. If a subluxation exists, there are specific tests or techniques which can be employed to determine if there is accompanying nerve interference. During a physical examination individuals having a displacement of the atlas vertebra often exhibit a "jump response" when even light pressure is applied to the neck area. Generally, children suffering from a misalignment of the atlas are very sensitive and this "jump response" is an involuntary neurological reaction due to severe cervical muscular tension.

Sessions:

Sessions are provided in the chiropractor's office. The number and frequency of sessions required for spinal subluxations associated with ADHD will vary depending upon the severity of the condition. Occasionally only one adjustment is necessary to correct the problem, but 10 to 20 or more sessions could be required. As with any treatment modality, the number of sessions will also depend upon the individual and how he or she responds to the treatment.

Although sessions are typically done once or twice a week, they may be more frequent if the problem is severe. The frequency of the sessions usually declines as the child improves. Once the problem is corrected, the child may or may not need to come back for occasional follow-up sessions. Also, periodic exams might be done to determine if there is a need for further care.

After the initial assessment, sessions are usually fairly quick and may last only 10 to 20 minutes. However, sessions may take more time if the chiropractor utilizes additional adjunct treatments in combination with the chiropractic adjustment.

Providers:

Doctors of Chiropractic complete several years of prerequisite undergraduate education and spend almost the same number of classroom hours at a fully-accredited chiropractic college as physicians do in medical schools. Included in their training is the appropriate use of highly sophisticated diagnostic equipment, laboratory procedures, and state of the art investigative technology. Before beginning practice, chiropractors must pass the National Boards as well as a licensing exam for the state in which they plan to practice. In addition, most states require them to attend clinical continuing education programs for annual licensure renewal.

Chiropractors are licensed in all 50 states of the United States to provide care to both children and adults. Doctors interested in providing the best possible care for children may likely belong to a chiropractic pediatric council and take regular continuing post-graduate courses in pediatrics. Some may even pursue a postgraduate degree in pediatrics.

The International Chiropractors Association has a Pediatrics Council to which many doctors belong. One of the functions of this Council is to provide regular updates in chiropractic pediatric care and to encourage its members to take advanced education courses in chiropractic pediatrics to improve their diagnostic and clinical skills. In fact, a Pediatric Certification is offered through the International Chiropractic Pediatric Association. This 120-hour curriculum offers techniques and protocols of care for children and pregnant women. The 10-module course goes above and beyond the training offered in chiropractic colleges.

Cost:

The cost for chiropractic care varies greatly. As with most services, it depends upon the area or region of the country in which the services are provided as well as who provides the services. Initial assessments will probably cost $100 or more. The cost could be substantially greater if x-rays and other medical tests are needed. The cost of the individual sessions will probably range from $20 to $100. This too may be substantially greater in some parts of the country or if adjunct treatments are utilized. Therefore, the overall cost for treatment could range from a few hundred to a few thousand dollars.

Unlike many other alternative therapies listed in this book, chiropractic care is usually covered by insurance. However, you will need to check with your insurance company to make sure this type of treatment is covered and to find out your co-payment since it may be more than co-payments for other medical procedures. Insurance will usually pay 75% to 80% of the charges leaving you with a co-payment of 20% to 25%. Usually support staff in a chiropractor's office can find out this information for you.

Most of the members of the International Chiropractic Pediatric Association (I.C.P.A.) offer complimentary consultations, allowing parents to meet with them in order to find out about chiropractic for their families and to discuss their individual needs. Be sure to ask your chiropractor if he or she offers this free service.

Research:
Summer Study

Seven children, ranging in age from 7 to 13, were involved in a summer study which examined the effectiveness of chiropractic manipulative therapy for reducing hyperactivity levels.[1] All of the children had clinical findings showing intervertebral subluxation (misalignment) complex, or spinal lesion. The study was conducted during summer vacation when the participants were home from school and off any stimulant medication they may have been previously taking. Pre-treatment data collection was done after the children had not taken any medication for a two-week period. The study was completed by mid-August.

One type of assessment measured the children's behavior using a wrist-watch type device to mechanically measure activity while the participants completed a 15-minute task, involving writing, which simulated schoolwork. During each visit to the chiropractor's office, prior to both the placebo and the actual intervention therapy, the motion recorder, or actometer, was placed on the child's non-dominant wrist and dominant ankle. The actual motion data used for each session was the average obtained for the arm and leg combined for an overall motor activity score. The researcher monitored these 15-minute sessions from a booth which was hidden from the children's view.

Other data collected were electrodermal tests to measure autonomic nervous system activity and chiropractic clinical evaluations to measure improvement in spinal biomechanics. Parental observations were also used for evaluation purposes.

Placebo care was administered prior to the chiropractic intervention. During the placebo treatment the chiropractor "pretended" to be treating the child with a detuned mechanical device adjusted down to zero thrust but with an audible "popping" sound. Non-specific contact points were used. The practitioner held the instrument between his index and middle finger so that it never actually touched the child. Since the instrument made a noise, it was perceived that the child assumed there was some benefit to the procedure. The child also received the same "gentle touch" before and after treatment as that used during the actual chiropractic intervention. In addition, the practitioner conversed with the child about hobbies, sports, summer vacation plans, and other topics, which was very similar to the dialogue used during the actual intervention sessions.

In reviewing the results of the study, all seven children showed at least some improvement in regard to the chiropractic measures assessed after the chiropractic intervention. Four of the seven children showed dramatic improvement in terms of the structural assessment of their spinal deviations. Four showed improvement in the level of autonomic activity. Five children showed a reduction in their average behavioral scores, as measured by the wrist-watch type device, after the chiropractic therapy. According to their parents, four of the children showed improvement in their behavior at home from the start of the study to the end of the treatment.

Although the behavioral improvement taken alone should only be considered suggestive, the strong inter-assessment agreement provides stronger evidence that a majority of the children did improve under specific chiropractic treatment.

Case Study #1: Diagnosed with ADHD at Age 2

One clinical study described the case of a five-year-old boy who had been diagnosed with ADHD at the age of two.[2] From age two to the time of chiropractic intervention at the age of five, the child's medical treatment consisted of his pediatrician prescribing Ritalin, Adderall, and Haldol. These medications offered little or no relief in regard to the child's inattentiveness, disruptive behavior, failure to complete tasks, forgetfulness, facial tics (which the parents observed began shortly after their son started taking Ritalin), and inappropriate outbursts at church and school.

At the age of five he was brought to a chiropractor to see if chiropractic care could help. The chiropractic examination and x-rays showed noticeable spinal distortion including a reversal of the normal neck curve indicative of subluxations. Chiropractic care was initiated and the child's progress was monitored.

Due to the severity of the condition and the limited time schedule of the child, a schedule of five visits per week was arranged. The child received 35 chiropractic treatments over an eight-week period. Around the 12th visit, the mother reported positive changes in her son's general behavior. Prior to this time, his behavior was very problematic.

After 27 chiropractic sessions, the child was taken to his medical doctor for a follow-up visit. At that time, his pediatrician reported that the child was no longer exhibiting symptoms of ADHD and concluded that the reduction was significant enough to discontinue the use of medications, which the child had been taking for three years.

The Clinical Biomechanics of Posture (CBP) protocol was used on the patient. It included mirror image adjustments, mirror image exercises, and mirror image extension-compression traction. In addition to adjustments and extension traction, all treatments included cryotherapy, or cold therapy, to reduce inflammation and reduce discomfort during traction.

This case study indicates that spinal correction using the CBP approach may have positive effects much greater than relief of musculoskeletal conditions. Indeed, during chiropractic care, the boy's facial tics disappeared and his behavior greatly improved. Altered spinal biomechanics associated with abnormal posture have a direct relationship to significant neurological stress and malfunction. Therefore, the researchers in this study suggest a possible connection between the correction of cervical kyphosis (rounding or curvature) in patients with ADHD and improvement in their ADHD symptoms.

Case Study #2: Nine-year-old with ADHD and Tourette's

Another case study dealt with a nine-year-old boy.[3] He had suffered from asthma and upper respiratory infections since infancy; headaches since age six; ADHD, Tourette's syndrome, depression, and insomnia since age seven; and neck pain since age eight. His medications included Albuterol, Depakote, Wellbutrin, and Adderall.

During the boy's initial chiropractic examination, evidence of a subluxation stemming from the upper cervical spine was found through radiographic and thermographic diagnostics. In addition, his mother reported that forceps had been used during the delivery.

Chiropractic manipulation employing an upper cervical technique was used to correct and stabilize the patient's upper neck injury. His condition was evaluated by thermographic scans as well as through observations by the doctor, the boy's parents, and the patient himself. After six weeks of therapy, all conditions (listed in the previous paragraph) were reported as no longer present. At this point, all medications, with the exception of a half-dose of Wellbutrin, were discontinued. At the end of five months, all symptoms continued to be absent for this patient.

Due to the onset of symptoms soon after the patient's birth, the immediate reduction in symptoms when treatment sessions were begun, and the total absence of symptoms within six weeks of undergoing chiropractic care, the chiropractor reporting this study indicated a connection between his patient's traumatic birth, his upper cervical subluxation, and his neurological conditions. Furthermore, the doctor suggested additional research investigating upper cervical trauma as a contributing factor to such conditions as ADHD, Tourette's syndrome, depression, insomnia, headaches, and asthma should be conducted.

Case Study #3: Nine-year-old with Hyperactivity, Short Attention Span, and Poor Impulse Control

This case study involved a nine-year-old girl whose primary ADHD symptoms were a short attention span, poor impulse control, and hyperactivity.[4] Her parents remarked that she had never been able to sit still or relax and that she had never taken naps. Every night she would wake up crying at least two or more times. Both her teacher and parents reported that she was struggling with reading and spelling and that her handwriting was illegible.

Through an x-ray of the cervical region, the chiropractor determined that this nine-year-old had a misalignment of the C-1 vertebra, or Atlas Subluxation Complex (ASC). A physical examination revealed a right leg deficiency when lying down, and a distorted right lower hip and shoulder while standing. She also exhibited a "jump response," where her whole body would jerk when slight pressure was applied to her neck.

After the first spinal adjustment, the girl's legs while lying down measured the same length, her hips and shoulders were even, and her sensitivity to being touched on the neck area was also reduced. A follow-up x-ray analysis showed a 50% reduction of the ASC. Her parents observed that she was more relaxed and had remained motionless for an extended period of time. In addition, she had been able to sleep through the night for the first time in her life.

At the end of the semester of school, this child had markedly improved her grades. Her reading level, which had been at the first grade level (1.5) when she began third grade, had increased to third grade level (3.5) in less than three months time. Her teacher noted that her handwriting had become legible and that, overall, she was both more poised and relaxed.

In questioning the child's parents on follow-up appointments, the chiropractor wanted to know if they had implemented any other changes for their daughter in regard to diet, nutrition, or activities she participated in which may have also influenced or affected her behavior or academic performance. He also asked if any changes or events had occurred in their family which may have been factors in the changes observed in his patient. According to the parents, everything, except for the ASC adjustments, had remained the same.

Other Case Studies

Brief descriptions of various other case studies are reported on the research link of the International Chiropractic Pediatric Association's website (www.icpa4kids.org/research/chiropractic/adhd.htm). Among those included are an eight-year-old girl with a history of epilepsy, bedwetting, and attention deficit disorder and a ten-year-old girl taking a daily dosage of 60 mg of Ritalin and having severe scoliosis.

Results:

Even though the duration of the "summer study" was short and the case studies were only about individual children, their findings suggest chiropractic manipulation may be a potentially valuable intervention for ADHD. If your child's ADHD symptoms are related to a spinal misalignment, you may expect initial improvements in one to ten sessions. If this subluxation is the only cause of the problem, you could expect your child to be completely normal with successful treatment. However, if a spinal subluxation is only a contributing factor but not the cause of the ADHD, then you might expect to see an improvement in ADHD symptoms but not a complete absence of them. In these cases, you should consider combining chiropractic care with other interventions.

Pros & cons:

Cautions: While chiropractic care may help if spinal misalignment is connected to your child's ADHD symptoms, it may not be 100% of the cause. Therefore, combining this with other supportive treatments may be more beneficial. Also, if a spinal misalignment is not a contributing factor, chiropractic treatment will not be effective.

Time: Due to the relatively short sessions of typically 10-20 minutes, your time commitment should not be a major issue. However, depending on the number of sessions your child may need, time could become a factor. Keep this in mind when looking for a chiropractor for your child.

Convenience: Since all 50 states and a majority of cities in the United States have practicing chiropractors, finding a local doctor should not present any problem. In fact, there are usually several in most towns.

Other: Since chiropractic care for ADHD may often produce better results when combined with other treatment modalities, using a chiropractor who also utilizes other treatment methods may be helpful.

Recommended reading and websites:

www.chiropractic.org
www.icpa4kids.org/research/chiropractic/adhd.htm
www.chiropracticresearch.org
www.icpa4kids.org—International Chiropractic Pediatric Association
www.nucca.com—National Upper Cervical Chiropractic Association

Contact information:

To find a pediatric chiropractor in your area, the I.C.P.A. website (www.icpa4kids.com/locator/index.php) has a Membership Referral Directory which can be searched by zip code, state, or city.

The National Directory of Chiropractic website (www.chirodirectory.com) also has listings where you can search by city, doctor's name, or county.

Another possibility would be to use MAPQUEST and enter "Chiropractors DC" in the "Find a Business category." In using this option, for example, we were able to find 149 chiropractors listed in our immediate area.

You may simply consult your local telephone directory. However, as with finding any other treatment provider, asking your friends, family, or coworkers may offer the best hope of finding the right one for your child. Since chiropractors are usually plentiful in most areas of the country, getting a personal recommendation should be fairly easy.

6

Massage Therapy

Names:

Massage Therapy
Massage
Bodywork
Somatic Therapy

What it is:

Massage therapy, often referred to as bodywork or somatic therapy, is the application of various techniques to the muscular structure and soft tissues of the human body. These techniques may include, but are not limited to, applying fixed or movable pressure, stroking, kneading, tapping, compression, vibration, friction, and rocking. Although massage therapists primarily use their hands in this application, sometimes their forearms, elbows, feet, or other devices are also used.

There are over 200 variations of massage, bodywork, and somatic therapies, and many practitioners employ multiple techniques. All techniques are utilized for the benefit of the musculoskeletal, circulatory-lymphatic, nervous, and other systems of the body.

With records dating back nearly 4,000 years documenting its use, massage therapy is recognized as one of the oldest methods of healing. It can be used on people of all ages, from newborns to seniors, and has been shown to have many physical and mental benefits.

How it works:

A typical full body massage will include work on the back, arms, legs, hands, feet, head, neck, and shoulders. The desired outcome of a therapy session is always discussed with the massage therapist. This conversation will guide the therapist in determining which body parts require massage, or where efforts may need to be specifically concentrated.

A massage or bodywork session usually takes place in a warm, comfortable, quiet room. Soft music may be played to assist in the relaxation process. The client will lie on a table, which has been especially designed for maximum comfort.

Traditionally most massage techniques are performed with the client unclothed. However, it is entirely up to the client (and you as the parent) as to what or how much your child should wear. Individuals should undress only to their comfort level. It is the therapist's job to see that the client is properly draped throughout the entire session. Only the particular area of the body being worked on is exposed while the therapist is giving the massage.

Frequently, a light oil or lotion is used to allow the client's muscles to be massaged without excessive friction of the skin. In addition, the oil helps to hydrate the skin. Massage works most effectively when the body is not resisting.

Many massage therapists practice a form of Swedish massage, which is often a baseline for them. In using such a technique, the therapist will begin with broad, flowing strokes that help calm the nervous system and relax exterior muscle tension. As the body becomes more relaxed, pressure will generally be increased to relax specific areas and relieve areas of muscular tension.

The use of massage therapy goes far beyond just relaxing the muscles. Massage therapy positively influences the overall health and well-being of the individual. It promotes a healing environment in the body which results in a large number of beneficial physical and psychological/mental responses. Some of these benefits related to ADHD are:

• increasing circulation, allowing the body to pump more oxygen and nutrients into tissues and vital organs,

• calming the nervous system,

• relaxing the whole body,

• promoting restful sleep, and

- improving concentration.[1]

Sessions:

Generally, massage sessions are 50 to 60 minutes long. However, they can be any length agreed upon between the client and the massage therapist. In two of the research studies mentioned in this chapter, positive results were achieved with only 15 and 20 minute massages.

The frequency of massage sessions also vary. In one of the research studies described in this chapter, massages were given daily. In the other study, massages were given twice a week.

Providers:

There are more than 100,000 massage therapists practicing in the United States at the present time. Although training requirements vary from state to state, an increasing number of schools and states are recommending massage therapy programs of at least 500 training hours. As of March 2004, 33 states have official massage licensing regulations.[2]

Depending upon the state, some massage practitioners are licensed by governmental authorities while others are not. In addition to certified or licensed massage therapists, there are professionals in other disciplines, such as physical therapists, who at times utilize massage as part of their treatment modality.

Cost:

The cost for massage therapy varies greatly. As with most services, it depends upon the area or region of the country in which the services are provided as well as who provides the services. One-hour massages may range from $25 to $75 or more. The cost of shorter massages, like the ones used in the research studies, will likely vary in price from $10 to $25.

If you follow a similar protocol to the one described in the research studies in this chapter, your child would be receiving a 15 to 20-minute massage for about 10 sessions. At an average cost of $20 per session, the total cost of this treatment would be approximately $200. Some massage therapists give discounts for multiple massages. Don't forget to ask about this discount as the research seems to indicate your child will need a number of massages, perhaps 10 or more, in a relatively short period of time.

The services of a massage therapist may be covered by health insurance when massage is prescribed by a chiropractor or osteopath. Also, as a general rule, therapies provided as part of a prescribed treatment by a physician or registered physical therapist are often covered. However, if your child is going to be receiving massage therapy for ADHD symptoms only, it will probably not be covered.

Research:
Touch Research Institute

The original Touch Research Institute (TRI), opened at the University of Miami School of Medicine in 1992, was the first center in the world specifically devoted to the study of touch. Since its beginning in the early 1990s, three additional TRI facilities have been opened. One location is in the Philippines, another is housed at the University of California at Los Angeles Medical School Pediatric Center, and a third location is at the University of Paris in France.[3]

The Touch Research Institutes have conducted more than 90 studies on the positive effects of massage therapy on various functions and medical conditions covering a wide range of age groups. These studies have been conducted by TRI researchers, along with their associates at other major universities such as Duke, Harvard, and the University of Maryland. If you go online to the TRI homepage (miami.edu/touch-research/index.html), you can access specific information regarding these various studies.

In fact, the two massage therapy and ADHD studies described next in this section were conducted by Touch Research Institute researchers. Both studies were worthy of being published in a peer-reviewed journal. As a side note, one of the co-authors of both articles is Dr. Tiffany Field, a well-known researcher in child mental health who has published several studies on the benefits of massage for infants. Dr. Field, who is a faculty member in the Department of Pediatrics, is the founder and director of the Touch Research Institute at the University of Miami School of Medicine.

Matched Study: Massage Therapy vs. Relaxation Therapy

In this study 28 boys were recruited from self-contained classrooms for emotionally disturbed adolescents. Participants, whose average age was 14.6 years, were randomly assigned to either the massage therapy or relaxation therapy group.[4]

The 14 boys in the massage therapy group received a 15-minute massage after school for 10 consecutive school days. The massage procedure consisted of moderate pressure and smooth strokes for five minutes each on the following body regions: (1) up and down the neck, (2) from the neck across the shoulders and back to the neck, and (3) from the neck to the waist and back to the neck along the spinal column. Each region received 30 back-and-forth strokes, at 10 seconds each, during its five-minute allotment.

Similarly, in the relaxation group, 14 boys participated in a 15-minute relaxation session after school for 10 consecutive school days. During each of these sessions, a therapist asked the adolescents to tense and relax the same parts of the body which were massaged each session in the massage therapy group.

Before and after assessments included the Happy Face Scale, completed by the boys themselves, and an assessment of fidgeting based on behaviors viewed by observers who were unaware of the participants' group assignments. In addition, other assessments included teachers' ratings of observed time on task in the classroom and on the Conners' Hyperactivity Scale, which identifies behavior problems in children ranging in age from 3 to 17 years old.

No significant before and after session changes were reported for the relaxation therapy group on any of the assessments. In contrast, at the end of the treatment, the massage group participants rated themselves as feeling happier and observers rated them as fidgeting less following the therapy sessions.

Additionally, the teachers of the massage group rated these students as spending more time on task and showing less hyperactive behavior in the classroom following the treatments. It is impressive to note that the teachers did not know which students had received which treatment and neither did the observers who rated them on their fidgety behavior.

In the discussion section of their article, the researchers pointed out that massage therapy could become a worthwhile tool in the management of ADHD, in conjunction with other presently used therapies. We believe it is important that studies such as this promising one be replicated, ideally with larger samples, to gain further knowledge regarding the value of massage therapy for use in the treatment of ADHD.

Matched Study: Massage Group vs. Wait-list Control Group

This study explored the effects of massage therapy on the behavioral, emotional, and physiological functioning in 30 ADHD children or adolescents who were receiving special education services.[5] Scores for all participants on both the hyperactivity and/or inattention subscales of the Conners' Teacher

Rating Scale confirmed they were displaying symptoms associated with ADHD at the beginning of the study. Participants were students attending a learning center for children and adolescents with academic and behavioral problems. The 30 children (24 boys, 6 girls) were between the ages of 7 and 18, with an average age of 13.

The participants were randomly assigned to either a massage group or a wait-list group in the study. Those in the massage group received two 20-minute massages per week for a total of nine treatment sessions. Each massage consisted of moderate-pressure stroking for four-minute intervals over the following body regions: (1) head/neck, (2) arms, (3) torso, (4) legs, and (5) back. Massages while lying on their backs lasted 10 minutes and included stroking of the forehead, gentle rocking (torso and legs), and continuous stretching of the Achilles tendon. Massages while in the "face down" position also lasted 10 minutes and included lateral lumbar stretches, neck squeezes, and kneading of the back.

Licensed massage therapists gave the massages in a large, quiet room located in the school building. Portable massage tables were used and all of the girls and boys remained fully clothed during each massage. The participants were told that the massages might help them relax. All therapy sessions were given at the same time each day (mid-afternoon) over the course of one month.

The children in the wait-list group did not receive any massages during the first month of the study and were told that not everyone was getting a massage because of the limited number of available massage therapists. Instead, the children in the control group were asked simply to relax for the same 20-minute time period twice each week. These children were told, however, that they would have an opportunity to experience the massage procedure on a voluntary basis during the following month.

Various assessments were taken at the first treatment session and again four weeks later at the eighth session. The assessments measured such things as: (1) mood state, (2) classroom behavior, and (3) stress level.

The results showed that the children in the massage group reported feeling happier after the first and eighth sessions. They also rated themselves as feeling better after the first and last day.

Teachers, who were unaware of which group the students were in, completed the Conners' Teacher Rating Scale at the first session and one month later for participants in both the massage and control groups. The following six factors from this 39-item scale were examined: hyperactivity, conduct problems, emotional-indulgent, anxious-passive, asocial, and daydream/attention problems. While there were reductions in all areas for the massage group, these reductions were especially significant in the areas of hyperactivity, anxious-passive behaviors, and daydreaming/inattention. Both the control and massage groups improved on the emotional-indulgent factor.

To measure stress, salivary samples were obtained. Each saliva sample was tested for cortisol, which is a hormone indicative of stress level. Samples were collected immediately before and 20 minutes after the control group and massage sessions on the assessment days, since cortisol response has a 20-minute lag time. No significant effects were reported for salivary cortisol in either group.

Soma Bodywork: A Case Study

Soma is a specific type of massage. It uses a protocol that includes deep tissue manipulation, movement training, dialogue between client and practitioner, journal keeping, repatterning, interpretation of drawings, and more.[6] Soma neuromuscular integration was developed in 1977. It has a 10-session structural format, with each session focusing on a particular area of the body. The sessions are designed for a cumulative effect, with each session building on the previous one.

The first work with ADHD children at the Soma Institute of Neuromuscular Integration in Buckley, Washington, began about 10 years ago when an eight-year-old boy was referred by a local physician.[7] Among the behaviors this child exhibited were the inability to follow directions, inability to work quietly, aggressiveness with other students and siblings, poor manners, and failure to accept responsibility for his behavior or actions. Prior to his referral, the boy had been seen by both school and private counselors, but with no apparent success.

This child reportedly enjoyed playing lots of computer games. The therapist viewed these games as very result-oriented, left-hemisphere activities. She described the boy as being bright, hating to be wrong, and liking to be alone. She reported that he had good mental awareness of his body, although he was uncomfortable in it most of the time.

During the first session, the therapist described her client as struggling with the idea of body awareness. As a result, she let him know that he could ask for the work to stop if it became too intense or invasive and this action gave him a sense of control.

When he returned for his second session, he reported that he had not been in any fights the previous week. Interestingly, the sessions were discontinued after the fourth week when the eight-year-old announced that he would "get better by myself now." Although this was not according to soma protocol and quite unusual, the therapist did not argue with the boy. Instead, she accepted and supported his decision. According to the therapist, children are not so "hard-wired," which means they are much easier to "fix."

It appears as though this eight-year-old did indeed get better, as he predicted he would do. Doing a follow-up on her former client approximately 10 years later, the therapist found him as a high school student no longer displaying ADHD symptoms.

This case study is discussed more in depth in the book *The Indigo Children*, by Lee Caroll and Jan Tober. According to the co-director of the Soma Institute of Neuromuscular Integration, she has offered soma bodywork to approximately 50 ADHD children in the last several years and has had only positive results.[8]

Massage Incorporated into Swedish Preschools and Grade Schools

Thousands of teachers of young children throughout Sweden have been trained to introduce massage into their classrooms over the past several years. Course participants learn how to massage children and how to teach children to massage each other, as well as how to integrate massage into everyday schoolwork. Some of the benefits of massage that have been reported from this work include the following:

- Children can concentrate more easily.
- Children become calmer and less aggressive.
- Children develop more empathy.
- Children fight less.[9]

Results:

According to the results of the two research studies described in this chapter, the following benefits were noted:

- improvement in mood
- increased time on task

- less hyperactive behavior
- fewer problem behaviors

One of the research projects documented positive results after 10 consecutive days of massage treatment with teachers noting positive changes within that timeframe. The other showed improvements were made within the 30 days in which the study was conducted. However, due to the lack of additional research, it is not known how soon one would expect to see the first signs of improvement or how long the improvements would last.

Pros & cons:

Cautions: Toxins are released from the soft tissues of the body during a massage. Consequently, it is recommended that an individual drink plenty of water following a massage. Drinking water is a safe and effective way of flushing the toxins out of the body.

Time: Depending upon what you want, the time for each session might range from 15 minutes to one hour. However, other factors you will want to consider are the number of sessions per week your child will be receiving as well as how much time is involved in traveling to and from the massage therapist's office.

Convenience: The convenience of this treatment method depends upon your proximity to a massage therapist. However, with more than 100,000 massage therapists practicing in the United States at the present time, you should be able to find one who is located near you. Also, some massage therapists will come to your home to provide their services. Although this would be the most convenient method, it would certainly add to the expense of this treatment option.

Other: Massaging your own child is worth looking into. At times, there are classes held where a massage therapist teaches parents how to properly massage their children. You can also request that your massage therapist teach you how to massage your child. It should be fairly easy to learn and doing your own massage therapy at home will help with both the financial aspect as well as the convenience of this therapy.

Most massage therapists are in practice with other massage therapists. While your child is receiving a massage, you may want to consider getting one for yourself at the same time.

Recommended reading and websites:

www.miami.edu/touch-research/index.html
www.massagetoday.com/archives

Contact information:

A good way to find a massage therapist is by searching your local yellow pages. If there is a massage school in your area, individuals there will likely know of a massage therapist near you. You might also ask your friends. Many people have been to a massage therapist or know of someone they could ask for a possible referral.

7

Acupuncture

Names:

Acupuncture
Acupuncture Therapy

What it is:

Begun over 2500 years ago in China, acupuncture is a technique in which a skilled practitioner inserts extremely fine needles into specific points on the human body to prevent or treat illness. It is a part of the holistic system of traditional Chinese medicine (TCM) which views health as a continuously changing flow of energy called Qi (pronounced "chee"). Acupuncture needles are most often inserted at specific locations on the skin called acupuncture points. These points are located on specific lines of the body called meridians. These meridians, also referred to as channels, are said to conduct Qi, the vital energy force of the body.

Pain or illness is believed to result from imbalances or blockages of the flow of Qi through the meridians. Acupuncture is traditionally thought to remove such blockages, restore the normal circulation of Qi, and improve overall health by promoting the balance of energy in the system. Therefore, simply stated, the goal of acupuncture is to restore health by improving the flow of Qi.

How it works:

The classic TCM explanation for how acupuncture works is that channels of energy (Qi) run in regular patterns through the human body and over its surface. These channels or meridians are like rivers flowing through the body irrigating and nourishing the tissues. An obstruction in the movement of these "rivers" is like a dam which backs up, creating imbalance and pain. Acupuncture needles can unblock the obstructions and reestablish the regular energy flow through the meridians.

A more Westernized medical explanation of acupuncture is that the stimulation of certain trigger points by acupuncture needles prompts the release of certain hormones and chemicals which reduce pain, regulate the body's endocrine system, and calm the nervous system. Inserting the needles at designated acupuncture points stimulates various sensory receptors which, in turn, stimulate nerves that transmit impulses to the hypothalamic-pituitary system at the base of the brain.

These hypothalamus-pituitary glands are responsible for releasing neurotransmitters and endorphins. The substances released as a result of acupuncture not only relax the whole body, they regulate serotonin in the brain. Increased circulation, decreased inflammation, relief from pain, and relief of muscle spasms are some of the physiological effects observed throughout the body when acupuncture is used.

According to the principles of traditional Chinese medicine (TCM) there are 14 primary channels or meridians which are associated with specific internal organs or organ systems. To remove blockages in these meridians, or to strengthen the flow of Qi, an acupuncturist inserts a number of tiny, flexible, sterile needles just under the surface of the skin. These needles are inserted at specific points called acupuncture points. There are literally thousands of these points located along the meridians.

Acupuncturists insert the needles in one of two ways. Needles may be inserted through a plastic tube which guides the needle into the skin or through traditional free-hand insertion. Almost all acupuncturists in the United States now use pre-sterilized, disposable needles which are used once and thrown away.

Although the needles may feel uncomfortable at times, they rarely hurt. Only about three times the thickness of a human hair, they are indeed very thin and much finer than the hypodermic needles used to give injections. They are solid, rather than hollow, which allows them to penetrate the skin easily with little resistance. Once the needles are inserted, the practitioner may twist them manually or send a weak electrical current through them to increase the energy flow. Depending upon the condition being treated, the needles may be left in place between 15 to 40 minutes. Some acupuncturists also use moxibustion, which involves the burning of specific herbs or other substances, near acupuncture points to accelerate the healing process.

Sessions:

Usually the first visit is the longest. This session will usually last about an hour to allow for a complete medical history and exam. During this visit your acupuncturist will observe your child, take your child's pulse, and ask various questions about your child's condition.

The practitioner will want to obtain as complete a picture as possible about your child's treatment needs. This holistic approach is typical of traditional Chinese medicine. It is wise to let the acupuncturist know about any other therapies and/or medications that are currently being used.

Follow-up sessions will typically last from 15 to 45 minutes, depending on the practitioner and the individual patient's needs. Generally, these visits will start with a few questions and a brief examination, followed by insertion of the needles. Sometimes other therapies, such as moxibustion or massage, are incorporated with the acupuncture treatment.

Individuals experience different sensations from acupuncture. Some describe a slight tingling "pins-and-needles" feeling while others may feel a little numbness or nothing at all. Most patients find the sessions relaxing, and it is not at all unusual for an individual to fall asleep during or immediately after a treatment.

Providers:

States vary in who is allowed to practice acupuncture. While some states license, certify, or register non-physician acupuncturists, other states limit the practice of acupuncture to physicians only.

The practice of acupuncture has become well established in the United States and Europe in the last 30 years. A practitioner who is licensed and credentialed may provide better care than one who is not. While a majority of states have established training standards for certification to practice acupuncture, not all states require acupuncturists to obtain a license to practice.

In states which require certification or licensure, professional acupuncturists must usually complete a minimum of three years of full-time study in a recognized acupuncture program or school. They must also pass a qualifying board exam. Most states use the examination developed by the National Commission for the Certification of Acupuncture and Oriental Medicine (NCCAOM).

Practitioners may be called Licensed Acupuncturists (L.Ac.or Lic.Ac.), Registered Acupuncturists (R.Ac.), or Certified Acupuncturists (C.Ac.), Acupuncturist (A.P.), or Doctor of Oriental Medicine (D.O.M). However, in each case, state licensure means an individual has met eligibility requirements established by the state to practice acupuncture and/or Oriental medicine. It is advisable, therefore, to check the American Association of Oriental Medicine (AAOM) website at www.aaom.org to learn about the specific regulations for your particular state.

Laws also vary by state regulating the practice of acupuncture by physicians. A referral list of medical doctors who practice acupuncture can be found on the American Academy of Medical Acupuncture's website (www. medicalacupuncture.org).

The National Acupuncture and Oriental Medicine Alliance (www. aomalliance.org) has two referral website links which you can access on its website as well. Friends and family members may also be a source of referrals.

Cost:

Costs will vary depending on your locale and the training and experience of the practitioner. The first session is typically longer and more expensive than subsequent treatments. Initial sessions with non-physician practitioners may range from $50 to $100. Follow-up sessions usually range from $25 to $50. If the practitioner is also a physician, the cost of treatment sessions will generally cost more.

Based upon the research discussed in this chapter, the children needed 60 sessions to achieve the positive results. If the sessions cost $25 each, the total cost would be around $1,500. With sessions costing $50, the cost would be approximately $3,000.

Insurance companies differ in their coverage, and these differences are affected by a variety of factors including state regulations, licensure of the provider, and whether or not medical supervision is required. Although you will probably find that most insurance companies do not cover this treatment for

ADHD, you will need to check with your insurance company to find out for certain.

Research:
Chinese Study Comparing Acupuncture Treatment to Ritalin

This study compared a group of 155 children (116 boys and 39 girls) treated with acupuncture to a control group of 58 children (46 boys and 12 girls) treated with Ritalin.[1] The participants, ranging in age from 5 to 15, were all diagnosed with ADHD according to the DSM-IV criteria.

A course of treatment for the acupuncture group consisted of five treatments per week for two weeks. Each treatment lasted approximately 30 minutes. A total of six courses of treatment were administered. The effects of the treatment were analyzed at the end of the six treatment courses (after three months) and again one month later.

The children in the control group were given 5 mg of Ritalin in the morning and 2.5 mg at lunch. If the dosage was not strong enough, the amount was increased to 10 mg in the morning and 5 mg at lunch. If even stronger dosages were required, the Ritalin was increased as needed for each child; however, the dosage never exceeded 30 mg daily. Similar to the acupuncture treatment, the effects of using Ritalin were analyzed at the end of three months. The effects of Ritalin were again assessed one month after the children stopped taking their medication.

The effects of both acupuncture and medication were analyzed according to the 18 diagnostic symptoms listed in the DSM-IV. Participants were considered "cured" if all 18 symptoms had basically disappeared. If five or more of the 18 symptoms were relieved, the treatment was considered to have demonstrated a "marked" effect. For children where two to four symptoms has been resolved, the treatment was assessed as having "some" effect. If no improvement in any symptoms was shown, the treatment was considered to have "no" effect.

The effectiveness of the two treatments did not differ significantly after three months. The treatment effect in the acupuncture group was 82.58% and the treatment effect for the control (or Ritalin) group was 87.9%. The treatment results are shown in the following table:

Group	Cured	Marked Effect	Some Effect	No Effect	Cases
Acupuncture	19 (12.3 %)	72 (46.4 %)	37 (23.9 %)	27 (17.4 %)	155
Ritalin	21 (24.1 %)	21 (36.2 %)	16 (27.6 %)	7 (12.1 %)	58

However, the differences between the two groups after the children had stopped taking either acupuncture treatments or stimulant medication for one month were significant. While the treatment effect in the acupuncture group remained relatively stable at 82.6%, the treatment effect in the Ritalin group decreased to only 32.8%. A majority of the children in the Ritalin group had regressed into the "no effect" category. The number of children in the "no effect" category for the acupuncture treatment remained unchanged. The specific treatment results were as follows:

Group	Cured	Marked Effect	Some Effect	No Effect	Cases
Acupuncture	12 (7.7 %)	53 (34.2 %)	63 (40.7 %)	27 (17.4 %)	155
Ritalin	2 (3.5 %)	5 (8.6 %)	12 (20.7 %)	39 (67.2 %)	58

A few children received some symptom relief from acupuncture in the first few weeks of treatment. However, there was a direct relationship between the number of treatment courses and the treatment effectiveness: the more treatments, the higher the treatment success. For example, after three treatment courses (or at the midpoint of the treatment), all symptoms had disappeared for only one child while 38 children experienced "marked" symptom relief, 45 children showed "some" relief, and 71 showed "no" symptom relief. (Notice how these numbers compare with what was experienced after the total three month treatment courses.)

The study also examined the relationship between the children's age and the effectiveness of the acupuncture treatment as well as the relationship between the children's ADHD subtype and the effectiveness of the acupuncture protocol. The acupuncture treatment was more effective in younger children, especially with those who were under the age of 12. The acupuncture protocol was most effective in the treatment of the hyperactive subtype.

(Remember the DSM-IV criteria identify the three ADHD subtypes as hyperactive, inattentive, and mixed.) Acupuncture was least effective in treating children with the inattentive subtype. The differences in the treatment effect between the different subtypes were statistically significant.

Results:

Acupuncture was more effective for younger children than for older children in this study. According to the researcher, the cerebrum in younger children is still developing at a much greater rate than in older children. After age 12, the cerebrum has already reached adult-level form and shape. Therefore, with older children the regulatory functions which acupuncture can exert seem to be more limited.

A small percentage of children received some symptom relief from acupuncture in the first few weeks of treatment. However, most children needed the full six treatment courses to show the maximum effect of the treatment. In addition, acupuncture appears to be significantly more effective with hyperactive behavior than with inattentive behavior.

Pros & cons:

Cautions: Acupuncture is not recommended for children under seven years of age. The study described above reported benefits for up to one month after the treatments were over but did not indicate if the benefits continued over a longer timeframe.

Time: This is a time intensive therapy as it appears you will need to go to the provider's office as many as five times per week for 12 weeks to receive these treatments. However, some acupuncturists may be able to provide this treatment on a less frequent basis. The frequency and number of sessions should be discussed with the acupuncturist.

Convenience: Acupuncture is now widespread in the United States and Europe so finding a provider in most mid-size or large towns should not be too difficult. However, you will probably not find too many providers in one town. When you consider the number of sessions, which you will need to go to the practitioner's office to obtain, finding an acupuncturist near your home or school will definitely be a plus.

Other: The thought of needles on the scalp (or elsewhere) may cause some initial apprehension on the part of both children and parents. Even though the treatment involves needles, acupuncture need not be at all painful if the needles are inserted correctly. Interestingly, according to the researcher's comments in the study, children identified with the hyperactive subtype tend not to be overly scared of needles and, therefore, are perhaps more willing to give acupuncture a try.

Recommended reading and websites:

www.aaom.org—American Association of Oriental Medicine
www.medicalacupuncture.org—American Academy of Medical Acupuncture
www.aomalliance.org—The National Acupuncture and Oriental Medicine Alliance

Contact information:

American Association of Oriental Medicine
909 22nd Street
Sacramento, CA 95816
Toll-free number: (866) 455-7999
Phone: (916) 443-4770
FAX: (916) 443-4766
Mailing Address: P.O. Box 162340
                 Sacramento, CA 95816
E-mail: info@aaom.org

American Academy of Medical Acupuncture
4929 Wilshire Boulevard
Suite 428
Los Angeles, CA 90010
Phone: (323) 937-5514
E-mail: JDOWDEN@prodigy.net

The National Acupuncture and Oriental Medicine Alliance
6405 43rd Avenue Ct. NW Ste. A
Gig Harbor, WA 98335

Phone: (253) 851-6896
FAX: (253) 851-6883
E-mail: info@aomalliance.com

8

Aromatherapy and Essential Oils

Names:

Aromatherapy
Essential Oils

What it is:

Aromatherapy is the use of plant oils, including essential oils, for an individual's psychological and physical well-being. Essential oils are highly concentrated aromatic extracts which are distilled from a variety of plant materials including grasses, leaves, flowers, needles, twigs, bark, roots, and fruit peels. Natural plant extracts are produced by steam distillation, cold press, solvent, and enzyme extraction depending on the nature of the plant.

Although the term "aromatherapy" was coined by a French chemist in 1928, the practice of using aromatherapy dates back thousands of years to the early civilizations of China, Egypt, Greece, and Rome. Indeed, records dating back to 4500 B.C. describe the use of balsamic aromatic substances for medical conditions and religious rituals.[1]

Contrary to their name, essential oils are not really "oily-feeling" at all. Although most essential oils are clear, some such as patchouli, orange, and lemongrass, are yellow or amber in color.

It is important to distinguish essential oils from perfume or fragrance oils. Where essential oils are derived from real plants, perfume oils are artificially created fragrances or contain artificial substances. Unlike essential oils, perfume or fragrance oils offer no therapeutic benefits.

Presently, 98% of essential oils produced are used in the perfume and cosmetic industry while only about 2% are being produced for therapeutic and medicinal applications. In recent years the growing resurgence to use more natural products, including essential oils, has been fueled partially by the increased availability of aromatherapy information both in books and over the Internet.[2]

How it works:

The ability of essential oils to act on both the mind and the body is what makes these oils unique among natural therapeutic treatment options. The therapeutic treatments using essential oils follow three different schools or models of application. In the English model, a small amount of essential oil is diluted in a vegetable oil and the body is massaged. The ingestion and undiluted topical application of essential oils is prescribed in the French model. The German model advocates the inhaling of essential oils.[3]

The three different schools of application demonstrate the versatility and potency of essential oils. In some cases, inhalation might be preferred over topical application while topical application may produce better results under other circumstances. However, in other cases, all three methods of application (topical, ingestion, and inhalation) may be considered interchangeable and may produce similar benefits.

The chemistry of essential oils is very complex. In fact, each one may consist of hundreds of different and unique chemical compounds. It is the distillation process, however, that makes essential oils so concentrated. Often it may require an entire plant or more to produce one individual drop of distilled essential oil.

The chemical constituents or components of essential oils have been compared to human blood since they have several properties in common. Both (1) fight infection, (2) contain hormone-like compounds, and (3) initiate regeneration. In addition, essential oils have a chemical structure which is similar to the one found in the cells and tissues of the human body. Because of this, essential oils are compatible with human protein, and, as a result, they are readily identified and accepted by the body.

Essential oils have the distinctive ability to penetrate cell membranes and diffuse throughout the blood and tissues. The structure of essential oils is very similar to the makeup of human cell membranes. Since the molecules of essential oils are quite small, their ability to penetrate into the cells is enhanced.

When the oil is inhaled, the micro droplets are carried to the limbic system of the brain, which is the processing center for reason, emotion, and smell, and to the hypothalamus, which is the hormone command center. The essential oil micro droplets are also carried to the lungs where they enter the circulatory system. When these oils are applied topically, such as to the feet, they can travel throughout the body in a matter of minutes.

Some essential oils contain high levels of the chemical components sesquiterpenes, which can dramatically increase oxygenation and activity in the brain. Other essential oils, because of their unique ingredients, tend to play an important role in hormonal secretion and in balancing mood and emotions.[4]

Sessions:

The only sessions involved with this type of treatment are when you apply or breathe the oils. In either case, it should only take a minute or two. This does not have to be done in any specified location, such as a provider's office, since it can easily be done at home or at school. Even though you may use the oils several times a day, the time it takes will be minimal.

Some people choose to breathe in the aroma while they sleep. To do this, one only needs to purchase a diffuser that plugs into the wall and disperses a small amount of the oil into the air while sleeping. Again, this process takes only a minute or two and is easily accomplished.

Providers:

There is no single discipline or provider that utilizes essential oils exclusively. Aromatherapy educational institutions usually offer a certificate or a diploma in aromatherapy to a variety of people interested in learning this technique. At the time of this writing, it appears as though no state offers a license or certification especially for aromatherapy.[5]

There are several terms associated with providers that utilize essential oils or aromatherapy. Generally speaking, an aromatherapist is an individual who has formal aromatherapy training and has been licensed in a "hands-on" field, such as massage, nursing, or cosmetology. An aromacologist or aromatherapy consultant, is someone with formal aromatherapy training but who is not licensed for any hands-on field. An aromacologist is not allowed to touch clients in states or countries where hands-on licensing is a requirement.

Finding an aromatherapist or aromacologist will make it easy for you to obtain the most appropriate oils for your child and to use them in the safest and most effective manner. However, these professionals may be difficult to find in many parts of the country.

Another way to obtain the oils and to get the information on how to best use them is to talk to someone in a store that sells them. Most places that sell the oils have someone who is well versed in their use. Health food stores are a good place to start looking for these products. If they do not sell them, they probably know of some place in your area that does.

One sure way of finding a provider is to become your own provider. By ordering the books in the recommended reading list, you can learn which products to get and how to safely use them. (Note that the first study reported under the research section in this chapter showed positive results for the children by simply breathing the vapors directly from the bottle three times a day. It does not get much simpler than that.)

If you choose this method, you might want to order the oils yourself. However, if ordering by mail or over the Internet, we recommend that you use a reputable company such as Young Living and not just buy essential oil products from anyone. If you choose Young Living, you can order the oils from one of their distributors or directly online over the Internet.

Cost:

This is one of the least expensive treatments listed in this book. There is usually no expensive provider cost, since most of the information needed will be supplied gladly by the person who is selling you the oils.

While some essential oils can be expensive, most of the oils that you might be interested in for your child are relatively inexpensive. You will probably find the cost ranging from $10-25 for a bottle which should last for a month or more. If ordered by mail, there will also be the customary shipping and handling costs. The only additional cost might be a book or two if you want to do it yourself or perhaps extra products like a diffuser.

Research:
Lavender and Rosemary with Adults

Forty adults were randomly assigned to either a lavender (considered a relaxing aroma) or rosemary (considered a stimulating aroma) treatment group.[6] Three drops of either oil were placed on a cotton swab and placed in a vial which participants held about three inches from their noses for three minutes while they were seated in a special massage chair. The treatment instructions for the 30 females and 10 males were simply to breathe normally and sit quietly with their eyes closed.

Following the treatment, the lavender group reported feeling more relaxed and less depressed. Their increased beta power after the treatment, as measured by their EEG activity, supports their self-reported increased relaxation state.

In contrast, the rosemary group reported feeling both more relaxed and more alert following the treatment. The decrease in their frontal alpha and beta bands, as measured by their EEG activity, would support this increase in alertness as well. The rosemary group also had lower anxiety scores.

While the lavender group performed the math computations faster and more accurately following the aromatherapy, the rosemary group was only faster and not more accurate. The researchers viewed the math difference between the groups as surprising since the lavender group did not show the enhanced alertness that the rosemary group displayed. However, they concluded that the lavender group may have simply been more relaxed and therefore better able to concentrate, as reflected in both their self-reporting and the EEG data.

Study Utilizing Three Essential Oils with ADHD Children

One study, conducted by a medical doctor, examined the effectiveness of essential oils in the treatment of 34 ADHD diagnosed children, ages 6 to 14.[7] None of the children were on medication. Sixteen subjects (11 boys and 5 girls) were in the control group while 18 subjects (12 boys and 6 girls) were in the treatment group. Within the treatment group, the participants were divided into three different groups with six individuals per group. For each of these three groups, one of three essential oils was randomly selected.

The three essential oils used in the study were cedarwood, lavender, and vetiver. Cedarwood was chosen because of its high sesquiterpene concentration, which improves oxygenation of the cells of the brain. Lavender, which has both a sedating as well as a stimulating action, was also chosen. It sedates part of the brain while at the same time stimulating the brain's limbic region. The third oil selected was vetiver, which calms and balances the nervous system in addition to stimulating the circulatory system.

Each child in the treatment group was given a glass bottle of the appropriate essential oil to administer at home. The treatment consisted of inhaling the oil three times a day, using a technique of holding the open bottle next to the nostrils and taking three deep inhalations. This procedure was followed for a period of 30 days.

At the beginning of the study, all children were assessed on the Test of Variables of Attention (TOVA) and on the ratio of their beta and theta brain waves, as measured by real-time EEG equipment. (Beta waves reflect those waves being produced when an individual is alert and/or performing a task while theta waves reflect the brain lacking focus or in a state of daydreaming, but awake.)

At the end of the 30 days of treatment, each child was again administered the TOVA test and was retested on the real-time EEG. Beta-theta ratios were again recorded.

Analysis of the data showed a significant improvement for the vetiver group from pre to post-treatment as compared to the control group. The use of vetiver improved the brain activity and reduced the symptoms of ADHD for this group. A similar result was seen with the cedarwood essential oil group, although not statistically significant. (The lack of statistical significance could be the result of the relatively small number of subjects in the study.) The group using lavender showed no apparent improvement after the treatment program.

The results would indicate that the essential oil vetiver proved to be the treatment of choice in this study. The researcher pointed out that he would not hesitate to recommend using vetiver in the treatment of children diagnosed as having ADHD and would even consider using cedarwood in situations where vetiver was not available or other cases in which vetiver might not be appropriate.

As a side note, the medical researcher in this study also received several letters from the parents indicating that their ADHD child's behavior at home had improved. In some of these letters, the parents also reported that their child's teacher had informed them of improved behavior and performance at school.

European Study on Oxygenation in the Brain

The previous study was the only one we found specifically dealing with ADHD and essential oils. However, in a study conducted in Europe, researchers found that sesquiterpenes found in essential oils such as vetiver, patchouli, cedarwood, sandalwood, and frankincense, can increase levels of oxygen in the brain by as much as 28%.[8] Such an increase in oxygen in the brain may lead to a increased activity level in the hypothalamus and limbic systems of the brain. Such heightened activity could likely have dramatic effects on emotions, learning, and attitude, as well as immune function, hormone balance, and energy levels.

Identified Oils for ADHD: Taking a Closer Look

Since both vetiver and cedarwood were mentioned in the two previous studies, we decided to consult the *Essential Oils Desk Reference Third Edition*, compiled by Essential Science Publishing, in order to share what it said about these two essential oils. Additionally, we have identified other essential oils mentioned in connection with ADHD in the *Desk Reference* and described their individual properties or characteristics.

Vetiver is labeled as an antiseptic, an antispasmodic, a relaxant, and as a circulatory stimulant under its medical properties. Specifically, ADHD is listed first in its "uses" category. Other uses for vetiver include anxiety, rheumatism/arthritis, depression, insomnia, and skin care. Under the "fragrant influence" section, it is described as psychologically grounding, calming, and stabilizing. In addition, reference is made to the previously cited clinical study that used vetiver with ADHD children.

According to the *Desk Reference*, cedarwood is labeled as combating hair loss, antibacterial, and as a lymphatic stimulant. ADHD is listed among its uses, although hair loss and arteriosclerosis are listed first. Under "fragrant influence," cedarwood is reported as stimulating to the limbic region of the brain, which is the center of emotions, as well as stimulating to the pineal gland, which releases melatonin. Cedarwood is also recognized for its calming and purifying properties.

In addition to vetiver and cedarwood, the following single oils are listed under the ADHD section: lavender, sandalwood, cardamom, peppermint, and ledum. Surprisingly, in cross-referencing, ADHD is only listed in the "uses" category for vetiver and cedarwood, which we have already discussed. ADHD is not listed under uses for lavender, sandalwood, cardamom, peppermint, and ledum.

However, cardamom is described as uplifting, refreshing, and invigorating while sandalwood, much like cedarwood, is said to be high in sesquiterpenes, which stimulate the pineal gland and the limbic region of the brain. Lavender, though not found to be effective in the ADHD study reported earlier in this section, was described as calming, relaxing, and balancing, both emotionally and physically.

Lavender, as described in the *Desk Reference*, has been documented to improve both concentration and mental acuity. A study by Japanese researchers is mentioned where improved mental accuracy and concentration were demonstrated when certain aromas, among them lavender, were diffused in an office environment and in a test taking situation.

In addition to single oils, the *Desk Reference* includes a list of several blend products for ADHD treatment. Among these blends is one product named Brain Power which contains cedarwood, sandalwood, frankincense, melissa, Australian blue cypress, lavender, and helichrysum.

Results:

Results should be seen fairly quickly. As noted in the research, improvements were made in the 30 days that the one ADHD study was conducted. However, due to the lack of additional research, it is not known how soon one would expect to see the first signs of improvement or how long the improvements would last.

Pros & cons:

Cautions: Children should only have the gentlest of oils at extremely low doses. No oils should be taken internally without first consulting with a qualified practitioner. If any oils are going to be applied directly on the skin, a skin patch test should be conducted prior to using any oil to ensure that no irritation develops. Some oils may need to be diluted before being applied to the skin. Never put essential oils into or near the eyes.

Time: One of the pros of this treatment is the time factor. Most of the time demands are in the beginning while you search to find a provider or to educate yourself on how to use these oils. Once this is done, the treatment sessions are very short and there should not be a need for numerous visits to a provider.

Convenience: This treatment method is very convenient. It takes very little time to do the treatments, the treatments can be done almost anywhere, and the oils can even be delivered to your home via mail. If you are using a professional provider, only very few visits are necessary and once you learn what to use and how to use it, you can easily do everything yourself.

One of the drawbacks is that the treatments may need to be done several times a day so remembering to do them might be an issue. Also traveling with the oils can be problematic, as they are sensitive to heat, sunlight, and x-ray machines (airport security).

Recommended reading and websites:

Essential Oils Desk Reference, 3rd edition, (2004), compiled by Essential Science Publishing, available at www.essentialscience.net

Reference Guide for Essential Oils, 8th edition, (2004), compiled by Connie & Alan Higley, available through Abundant Health at www.abundant-health4u.com

www.youngliving.us—Young Living—a multi-level marketing company that sells essential oils

www.abundant-health4u.com—Abundant Health—a resource for books, educational material, and other products involved in properly utilizing essential oils

www.essentialscience.net—a resource for books, educational material, and other products involved in properly using essential oils

www.youngliving.org/LSL—if you can not find a provider of this product in your area, you can order essential oils from this address

Contact information:

Since there is no one particular discipline that is the primary provider of essential oils, you might begin by searching for either an aromatherapy practitioner or an establishment that sells essential oils. A good place to start would be in your local yellow pages under such headings as "aromatherapy," "aromatherapists," "aromatherapy consultants," "aromacologists," "holistic medicine," "alternative medicine," or "health food." Paying a visit or phoning these individuals or establishments may supply you with a provider of essential oils in your area.

Another option is to call local massage therapists. Frequently, they will know about or have someone on-site who sells essential oils. A final option would be to use the websites listed above to order your own oils and information as described in the provider section of this chapter.

9

Relaxation Training, Meditation, and Yoga

All of the techniques or treatments described in this chapter have a mind-body connection. What is the mind-body connection and how does it work? When we experience an emotion, it generates a feeling which turns into a physical sensation. For example, if you are watching a horror movie, you feel frightened and then get a chill up your spine. In this particular case you are getting a negative suggestion through your eyes and ears which produces a feeling of fear. This emotion of fear turns into the physical sensation of chills up your spine.

Another example of this mind-body connection happens if you imagine taking a bite out of a lemon. Just think about the following: picking up a bright yellow lemon, holding it to your mouth, and taking a bite out of it just as you would an apple. The effect is even more pronounced if you imagine the acidic lemon juice squirting in your mouth as you chew bitter rind and swallow it. Yuck!

When a person is physically relaxed, mental relaxation follows, and when a person is mentally relaxed, physical relaxation follows. Relaxation training can alleviate anxiety because whenever you relax either the mind or the body, both the mind and the body become relaxed.

Relaxation Training

Names:

Relaxation Training
Progressive Muscle Relaxation
Controlled Breathing
Visualization

What it is:

Relaxation training is a treatment approach which seeks to develop an individual's ability to consciously relax the muscles of the body at will. Its purpose is to identify and then lessen tension during normal daily activities, as well as prior to or during stressful situations.

Most relaxation procedures currently in use in the United States are derived from the work of Edmund Jacobson, who in the 1920s and 1930s, pioneered the field by developing progressive muscle relaxation exercises. Although reduced muscle tension is often accomplished by using progressive muscle relaxation procedures, it can also be achieved through a number of other techniques and procedures, such as deep or controlled breathing, visualization, or meditation.

Progressive muscle relaxation is a technique in which the body's major muscle groups are alternately tensed and relaxed. The process can proceed from the head to the feet or in a reverse manner starting with the feet. An individual tenses and relaxes the muscles in the forehead, eyes, jaws, neck, shoulders, upper back, biceps, forearms, hands, abdomen, groin, legs, hips, thighs, buttocks, calves, and feet. By sitting and alternately tensing and relaxing major muscle groups for brief periods of time, individuals learn to become more aware of when their muscles are tense or relaxed.

Deep or controlled breathing is based on the observation that many of us breathe shallowly or irregularly when we are anxious or tense. These breathing patterns lead to an imbalance of oxygen and carbon dioxide in the body, which can cause symptoms of anxiety. Deep breathing plays an important part in yoga and in other Eastern relaxation techniques as well.

Visualization, or mental imagery, involves the use of pleasant scenes of peaceful situations to promote relaxation. It refers to an individual's ability to picture soothing, restful images in the mind.

How it works:

The basic idea behind progressive muscle relaxation is to systematically train various groups of muscles. These exercises involve the tensing and releasing of muscle groups in a prescribed sequence, leading to an increased awareness of the resulting sensations of tension and relaxation.

All exercises are done sitting in an upright position. The eyes may be closed or open while performing the training. During the initial training sessions, each group of muscles (forearm, upper arm, etc.) is exercised separately. Each muscle group is tensed for a short period of time (from 2 to 5 seconds) and then relaxed for a longer period of time (from 15 to 30 seconds). This same procedure is then repeated. After the individual has alternately tensed and relaxed, each muscle group is relaxed without tensing. Later these exercises are combined so that at the end one should be able to relax the whole body at once.

It is estimated that the whole procedure should last about 20 to 25 minutes. However, the length of time will vary with the age, ability, and receptiveness of the child. Some children will need considerable guidance and prompting. Between these training lessons, regular daily practice is recommended.

At the conclusion of the progressive relaxation exercise, deep breathing is recommended. Individuals should breathe in deeply, moving their fingers and toes. Next, they should breathe in deeply and stretch. Finally, they should breathe deeply and open their eyes if they were previously closed.

Since different individuals carry muscle tension in different parts of their bodies, the particular areas that need emphasis will vary from person to person. Relaxation is a skill that can be developed much like playing the piano or throwing a ball. Repeated practice of any relaxation method will create even deeper levels of relaxation. The more one practices, the greater the development of the skill.

Controlled breathing should be practiced for a minimum of four minutes, because this is approximately how long it takes to restore the balance of oxygen and carbon dioxide in the body. The balancing works more effectively if you breathe in and out deeply an equal amount of time.

There are various simple exercises to illustrate how deep breathing works. For example, if a person puts one hand on the upper chest and the other hand on the stomach, the hand on the stomach moves out as the individual breathes in. Another exercise involves breathing in to a slow count of four and out to a slow count of four. If this is done for at least four minutes, the person will become more relaxed. Whether one breathes through the nose or mouth does not matter. What is important is to be comfortable, breathe gently, and not to take large gulps of air.

Visualization involves actively picturing scenes that are tranquil and relaxing to the individual. Scenes may be actual places a person knows which feel safe and relaxing, or they may be scenes a person creates to be peaceful, safe, and relaxing. The specific scene is not as important as how the image actually makes the individual feel.

As a general rule, the more senses which can be incorporated into the image, the more relaxing visualization is likely to be. If individuals can imagine the sounds, smells, tastes, and tactile sensations as well as the visual components of a scene, they will be more likely to improve their ability to relax. For example, if they can imagine themselves walking along a sandy, tropical beach, they may want to focus their attention on the waves lapping, the sunlight shimmering on the water, the smell of flowers or the salt air, the blueness of the water, and the warm breeze as it touches their skin. Each one of the senses can contribute to the experience of relaxation and comfort.

Once trained in imagery, the individual must learn to shift from unpleasant images to those which promote or induce relaxation. Relaxation tapes can often be used to guide mental imagery or visualization.

Sessions:

Most individuals are able to learn some relaxation exercises in as little as one 20-30 minute session. Practicing the exercises takes about the same amount of time. However, the more they are practiced, the quicker the child is able to achieve the desired relaxed state.

Providers:

Since many of these exercises are fairly easy to do, most people are able to learn them from following instructions in books, audio tapes, video tapes, DVDs, etc. However, if you want to learn them from a provider, almost any type of mental health therapist can teach them to your child.

Cost:

The cost is very low if books or tapes are used to teach these procedures as they can be purchased for as little as $10 to $25. If a mental health therapist or other trained professional teaches the exercise, they will probably charge their normal hourly rate which could be $50 to $100 or more. However, since only one or two sessions are usually needed, this cost too is minimal.

Research:
Overview

Since the 1970s numerous research studies have been conducted investigating the effectiveness of relaxation training with ADHD children. In several studies, muscle tension was reduced by some form of relaxation training. Using parent and teacher behavioral ratings, a majority of studies reported improved behavior, while a few cited no differences or mixed results. Similarly, cognitive performance measures were improved in several studies as well, although mixed results and no improvement were shown in others. Additionally, improvements in self-concept were reported in some of the research findings.

While there is some inconsistency, overall the evidence of the effectiveness of relaxation training with hyperactivity is promising. Not wishing to have the reader "wade" through all of the various studies, we have included only a small sampling to provide some idea of the variety of research which has been done in this area.

Group Relaxation Training and Large Muscle Exercise Effects on ADHD

Thirty-four hyperactive first and second graders were randomly assigned to one of three groups: (1) a relaxation group, (2) a large muscle exercise group, or (3) a control group.[1] None of the participants, who were all boys, had been on any medication for their hyperactivity for at least three years.

Before and after assessments were the Nowicki-Strickland Locus of Control Scale (LCS) and the Matching Familiar Figures Test (MFFT). High scores on the LCS correlate negatively with achievement. The MFFT measures both attention to visual detail and impulsivity.

The first group treatment session was held one week after the initial assessments were completed. Two more group treatment sessions occurred at one-week intervals. Treatment assessments were given again one week after the last group session. All assessments were done individually.

For the relaxation group (12 boys) and the large muscle exercise group (11 boys), instruction at each of the sessions was identical. The only difference was that parental involvement was an additional component of the large muscle group. Parental involvement, however, varied greatly in the study and the researchers were disappointed in the degree of involvement.

At each session the children were first given five minutes to get settled. The next 10 minutes focused on the relaxation training with the instructor first demonstrating each segment and providing feedback as the children underwent the training themselves. This segment was followed by 10 minutes of large muscle exercise. Finally, each session was concluded with a repetition of the deep breathing exercise. This was completed while the children were resting and sitting quietly. The deep breathing was implemented throughout the large muscle exercise segment. The children were taught to "inhale up" (as in lifting their leg or arm) and to "exhale down" (as in lowering their leg or arm).

Treatment in the control group consisted of the 11 children listening to narrated versions of children's stories. These stories were selected for their "neutral" qualities, since they did not have an arousal or relaxing effect on the participants.

The results of this study indicated that both the relaxation group and the large muscle exercise groups demonstrated significantly higher attention to task scores and lower impulsivity scores, as measured by the MFFT, than the control group. Participants in the treatment group with the parental involvement component exhibited more internal (lower) locus of control at the end of the study than the other two groups.

Discussion

The findings provide some evidence that it is possible to teach young children a technique by which they can modify their own behavior in a relatively short timeframe. Indeed, the reporting of positive results after only three weeks of training was encouraging.

Using Relaxation and Exercise for Hyperactivity and Impulsivity

This study compared relaxation and exercise programs with attention-placebo, no-treatment, and non-hyperactive control groups.[2] Placebo means that the person received what he or she thought was the actual treatment but was really something that would have no effect.

Eight 3rd grade teachers rated their students' classroom behavior on a hyperactivity questionnaire modeled after the Conners' rating scale. The 24 students, who were all boys, with the highest scores (those displaying the most "hyperactive and impulsive" behaviors) were randomly assigned to one of four treatment groups: (1) muscle relaxation, (2) large muscle exercise, (3) attention-placebo control, and (4) no-treatment control. A fifth group included one boy from each classroom who scored in the bottom 25% of his class on hyper-active behaviors and whose performance in school was matched with a class-mate assigned to the no-treatment control group.

Participants assigned to the muscle relaxation, large muscle exercise, and attention-placebo control groups received five individual 20-minute training sessions over a period of three weeks. The first two sessions involved (a) pro-gressive relaxation training, (b) strenuous exercise, or (c) using modeling clay to make objects. The task of making objects with clay was chosen for the attention-placebo group since it was considered neither especially rewarding nor boring.

For the last three sessions, participants spent the first 10 minutes relaxing, exercising, or playing with clay, depending on their assigned treatment group. During the last 10 minutes of these sessions, the children were asked to solve card games or mazes which required attention and concentration skills. While those in the relaxation group were encouraged to practice their muscle relax-ation techniques during the game playing activities, those boys in the exercise group were instructed to engage in 30 seconds of doing push-ups at regular intervals. Those individuals in the other groups were given no intervention strategies during these sessions.

A week following the completion of the training programs, the Matching Familiar Figures Test (MFFT) and a shortened version of the Continuous Performance Test were individually administered to all participants. Those in the relaxation group were encouraged to use relaxation for a minute or two before each test while those in the exercise group were directed to do push-ups and sit-ups for a minute or two before each test. In contrast, individuals assigned to the remaining groups were simply given a minute or two of unstructured time between tests.

Results showed that accuracy on the MFFT, which measures impulsivity and attention to visual detail, was significantly higher for the relaxation group, the exercise group, and the non-hyperactive control group as compared to the no-treatment control group. No significant differences were found on the shortened version of the Continuous Performance Test. The researchers noted, however, that using the abbreviated version may have biased the results.

Discussion

The findings of this study suggest the effectiveness of both progressive relax-ation techniques and large muscle exercises in treating impulsive, hyperactive children. However, the effects of relaxation and exercise training were potentially confounded by the brief relaxation or exercise period just before testing. The researchers acknowledged the possibility exists that the one or two minutes of relaxation and exercise alone before the MFFT was administered may have yielded the observed effects.

The results for the relaxation training were viewed as promising by the researchers. They reported, however, that the skill or proficiency level among the children appeared to differ markedly during the relaxation training sessions. While several children demonstrated an appropriate skill level, they noted that a few children's behaviors were more characteristic of restlessness than relaxation. Shifting positions and opening and closing their eyes were some of the behaviors exhibited by those who were more restless.

Examining individual test results revealed that those participants who appeared less proficient in relaxation techniques generally performed less well on the test measures. One recommendation suggested by the researchers was that some children might feasibly profit from longer and more individualized training.

Results:

The results of both research studies show promise and indicate that teaching relaxation methods to children with ADHD would be worthwhile.

Pros & cons:

Cautions: None

Time: With sessions taking as little as 20 to 30 minutes, it takes very little time to both learn and practice these techniques.

Convenience: This is one of the most convenient treatment methods since most of these exercises can be both learned and practiced almost anywhere.

Other: Due to the low cost, lack of any cautions, and potential benefits, this intervention would be worth considering for almost any child with ADHD.

Recommended reading and websites:

There are numerous books and tapes on this subject. They can be easily found at your local bookstore or from many discount suppliers of books and tapes. Your public library may also be a source of some materials on this subject.

Contact information:

If you plan to contact a mental health professional to provide this service, your local phone book will provide you with numerous listings. However, as with all providers, recommendations from friends or family members who have received services from someone may be your best source.

Meditation

Names:

Meditation
Mindfulness Meditation
Concentrative Meditation

What is it:

Broadly defined, meditation is any activity that keeps an individual's attention pleasantly anchored in the present moment in time. All meditative practices have one thing in common—they all focus on quieting the busy mind. When a person's mind is calm and focused in the present, it is not reacting to past memories or being preoccupied with future plans.

Basically, all meditation techniques can be grouped into either concentrative meditation or mindfulness meditation. Concentrative meditation focuses a person's attention on breathing, an image, or a mantra (sound), in order to quiet the mind and allow more awareness and clarity to emerge. You might compare this to a zoom lens on a camera; the individual is narrowing his or her focus to a selected field. In its simplest form, concentrative meditation is when a person is sitting quietly and focusing attention on breathing.

Mindfulness meditation can be compared to a wide-angle lens. Rather than narrowing your focus as in concentrative meditation, you will actually become more aware of the entire field. Your mind is opened to become aware of the continuously passing parade of sensations, feelings, images, thoughts, sounds, and smells you are experiencing. In mindfulness meditation, one sits quietly and simply witnesses whatever is going through the mind, not reacting or becoming involved with memories, thoughts, worries, or images. By not becoming involved, one is gaining a calmer, clearer, and more non-reactive state of mind.

How it works:

One of the primary ways of quieting the mind is by using one's breath. Meditation practitioners, as well as yoga instructors, believe there is a direct correlation between an individual's breath and an individual's state of mind. For example, when one is anxious, frightened or distracted, breathing will tend to be shallow, rapid, and uneven. In contrast, when the mind is calm, focused, and composed, breathing will tend to be slow, deep, and regular. Focusing your mind on the continuous rhythm of inhaling and exhaling provides a natural method for meditating. As you become focused on your breathing, your mind becomes absorbed in the rhythm of inhalation and exhalation. Consequently, your breathing will become slower and deeper, and your mind will become calmer and more aware.

The practice of meditation can bring about a healthy state of relaxation by reducing heart rate, respiration rate, and pulse rate. There is also a decrease in cortisol, a major stress hormone produced by the body. During meditation the brain produces increased alpha waves which are linked with deep relaxation and mental alertness. The alpha waves produced during meditation are more intense than those produced during sleep, making meditation highly beneficial for reversing the damaging effects of stress.

Sessions:

Most of the benefits derived from practicing meditation can be obtained by meditating for a relatively short period of time. While learning to meditate, your child may want to start out by trying it for only 5 to15 minutes once or twice a day. Building up to a 20-minute session should produce substantial benefits as noted in the research in this chapter. You may have heard about some people who meditate for an hour or more each day; however, this length of time should not be necessary for your child.

Providers:

There are many techniques of meditation, but it is doubtful that any particular one is going to be superior to the others as far as reducing the symptoms of ADHD. Therefore, in finding a source to learn meditation, you might want to consider your children learning mediation from video tapes, audio tapes, CDs, or even books rather than feeling that they have to learn a particular technique from a certified provider that sometimes is very expensive. Providers, books, tapes, and CDs that teach mediation methods can be found in the recommended reading and websites section at the end of this chapter.

Cost:

Learning meditation from books, audiotapes, videotapes, or CDs is very affordable and the only cost is that of purchasing the book or tapes. This expense will vary depending upon what you buy, but should be somewhere between $25 and $100.

If you use a certified provider for this service, be sure and discuss the cost with that individual since the charges could be as much as $2,500 or more for the training. Generally, insurance will not cover the cost associated with meditation.

Research:
Comparison of Meditation, Muscle Relaxation, and Control Group on ADHD

Twenty-four boys, who were diagnosed as having ADHD, were randomly assigned to one of three groups: (1) a meditation training group, (2) a progressive muscle relaxation group, and (3) a waiting list control group.[3] The children ranged in age from 7 to 12.

Those assigned to the meditation training group met individually with the researcher for 20 minutes twice weekly for the four-week treatment period. During each training session, the children sat with their eyes closed and took deep, slow breaths. Following the researcher's example, the children repeated "ahnam," a Sanskrit word meaning nameless, aloud. The periods of repeating the word gradually increased from two to eight minutes.

Children in the muscle relaxation group met individually with the researcher for the same amount of time each week as the meditation group. They followed a tension-relaxation cycle which included the following: hands, forearms, biceps, triceps, shoulders, stomach, thighs, and legs. They were also taught a deep breathing technique to be used both before and after the tension-relaxation exercises. The time period of this group's relaxation exercises gradually increased from two to eight minutes as well.

Participants in both the meditation and the relaxation groups were asked to practice at least three times per week at home. This resulted in a total of five sessions a week. Additionally, following the second week of training, the parents were seen individually for one session to learn the meditation procedure and the relaxation technique themselves so they could act as resources for their children.

In contrast, at the beginning of the study those in the control group were simply told they would begin their relaxation training in about four weeks. Otherwise, during the study's time frame, they received no other treatment.

All participants were assessed on the following measures: Matching Familiar Figures Test (MFFT), Fruit Distraction Test (FDT), Nowicki-Strickland Locus of Control Scale (LCS), Conners' Abbreviated Parent-Teacher Questionnaire (PTQ), and Werry-Weiss-Peters Activity Scale (WWPAS). These assessments were given individually one week prior to the beginning of the study and again in the week following the last treatment session.

Results indicated that both the meditation and relaxation groups showed significant decreases in levels of impulsivity as measured by their MFFT scores. Parent rating scales (PTQ) reflected a significant improvement in the behavior of the children in both the meditation and relaxation groups as well.

Both the meditation and relaxation groups showed significant improvement on their WWPAS scores, which measured activity level in specific situations. Although both groups demonstrated significant gains, the scores of the meditation group in particular reflected marked improvement in the "homework" and "behavior during meals" items.

Pre and post-test comparisons on the FDT (used to determine how well an individual can attend to relevant information) revealed that only the meditation group showed a significant decrease in the number of errors. No significant changes occurred for any of the three groups regarding locus on control.

Discussion

Parents in the study offered several supportive comments regarding their child's behavior. Their observations included an increased ability to sit quietly, to complete homework assignments, and to focus attention. Some parents were relieved to have a "tool" to use to enable their child to calm down and be more in control. Those parents who were fearful or reluctant to have their child on medication were pleased to have a non-medical intervention option.

Additionally, various encouraging and positive comments were voiced by the participants themselves regarding the meditation technique. One child said he felt sleepy, calm, and relaxed all at the same time. Another boy described the technique as a "miracle." He noted that he had never stayed so calm for so long in his whole life. A third boy focused on how it had helped him in school. He could ignore the distractions around him and focus on getting his work done. One other child reported that he had been able to make up over 20 homework assignments since he could finally sit down and work without feeling so restless and fidgety.

The researcher also noted that several of the children reported they had used the meditation technique to help them sleep at night. Interestingly, one boy who had repeatedly hit his head against a pillow before falling asleep found the technique so helpful that his head banging behavior was eliminated.

Sahaja Yoga Meditation as Family Treatment Program

This Australian study examined meditation as a family treatment method for ADHD children, using the techniques of Sahaja Yoga Meditation (SYM).[4] Parents participated with their children in a six-week program of twice-weekly clinic sessions and regular meditation as home. Forty-eight children (41 boys, 7 girls), including four sets of siblings, participated. A majority of the children were receiving medication. The children ranged in age from 4 to 12.

During the first three weeks, the clinical sessions consisted of guided meditation sessions, with parents attending one group and children attending a separate group. During these sessions instructors helped parents and children to learn techniques to achieve a state of thoughtless awareness. Instructors further directed the participants to become aware of this state within themselves by becoming silent and focusing their attention inward. Additionally, parents were asked to conduct shorter meditation sessions at home twice daily.

The clinical sessions, which were 90 minutes in length, were held in large meeting rooms in a hospital setting. Each 90-minute session consisted of two periods of meditation each lasting between 5 and 15 minutes, information about how to meditate, and a sharing time.

During the second half of the study, one of the weekly clinical sessions was conducted as a joint parent-child meditation. This allowed instructors to train the parent in guiding the child's meditation. As a result, parents and their children were asked to meditate regularly at home during weeks 4 to 6 and to record their progress in a diary. This diary was checked each week to courage compliance.

Testing was done at the beginning of the study (week 1), at the midway point of the program (week 3), and at the end of the program (week 6) using several evaluation methods. At each of these points, parents were asked to complete the following assessments regarding their children: rating scale on their child's ADHD symptoms (Conners' 11-item checklist), questionnaire on benefits of treatment, report on any changes in medication, and 13-item self-esteem questionnaire. In addition, parents completed two assessments on themselves. These included reporting on whether the meditation program had been beneficial to them and completing a 30-item Child-Parent Relationship Scale (CPRS) which assessed the quality of the parent-child relationship.

Individual interviews were conducted with each child at the end of the six-week meditation program. Questions asked during these audio-taped sessions focused on the following: the children's experiences, whether they liked meditation, what they liked about it, whether they felt it had been helpful to them, and how meditation had actually been useful or beneficial.

Thirty-five of the 48 participants completed the full six-week program. Complete data were collected on 26 children and results reflect the findings on these children only.

Results showed improvements in the children's ADHD behaviors as measured by the Conners' Parental Rating Scale. Improvements in self-esteem and the quality of the parent-child relationship were also identified.

Parents reported a reduction in medication in several cases. Of the 20 children who were receiving medication when they began the meditation program, 11 were able to reduce their medication during the course of the program. Interestingly, the improvement in ADHD symptoms was significantly greater for those 11 children than for the 9 children who had maintained the same level of medication. According to the authors of the study, this finding suggests that the SYM treatment not only contributed to the reduction in ADHD behavior scores, but also had the additional benefit of helping the children manage their behavior with a reduced level of medication. Children in post-treatment interviews also viewed stopping or reducing their medication as one of the positive outcomes of the program.

Other information gained from the individual interviews showed that the children had a positive attitude toward the meditative treatment and described numerous benefits they had gained by practicing SYM. Some of the benefits the children reported included the following: getting to sleep more easily, focusing better at school, concentrating more easily, having fewer social problems, being less panicky, feeling calmer, and being more relaxed.

The parents' assessment of the results agreed with the viewpoints of the children. In fact, 92% of the parents agreed that their child had definitely benefited from the meditation program. Among the benefits parents rated highly were: more confident, improved sleep patterns, more cooperative, less difficulty with the teacher, more able to manage schoolwork, more able to manage homework, and more positive about going to school.

The vast majority of the parents (92%) saw the program as being personally beneficial as well. Benefits receiving the highest rating included: more able to manage stress, less stress, happier, more able to manage anger, and less angry. When asked to rate the extent to which they felt that SYM had benefited their relationship with their child, parents rated the following items highest: more open communication, less exhausting, more able to manage conflict, and less conflict.

Discussion

This is the first study conducted to examine the effect of Sahaja Yoga Meditation as a treatment for ADHD. Its aim was to investigate SYM as an additional family-oriented treatment in conjunction with any conventional medical treatment being received by the children.

While the positive results of this trial program were consistent and appear promising, the study is not without its limitations. First, the small number of children for whom complete data were available is a concern; the study had a relatively high drop-out rate. The lack of a formal control group is another concern. There was, however, a "waiting list" of children that acted like a quasi-control group. Baseline ADHD scores were collected on this group at recruitment and at week 1 of the treatment program. Their ADHD scores, which were taken again at the end of the six-week period, did not improve.

The preliminary findings of this study provide initial evidence of the benefits of Sahaja Yoga Meditation in alleviating the behavioral symptoms of ADHD children. The positive effects are confirmed through parental reports and through the children themselves. According to the children, the benefits extended beyond their home environment into their classrooms.

Results:

The results of both studies discussed above indicate that meditation appears to be an effective intervention for children diagnosed as having ADHD. The findings of the first study also seem to support the usefulness of a muscle relaxation approach in treating ADHD.

The benefits also appear to become evident fairly quickly as both studies reported positive results within the timeframes of the studies which were only four and six weeks in duration.

Pros & cons:

Cautions: While meditation is not in itself a religious practice, there are some forms of meditation that are closely connected with spiritual teachings. You may want to review the teaching material or visit with the provider of this service before your child begins. This would ensure that if there were any spiritual connections with the training, that they are congruent with your own belief system.

Time: Meditation, especially for children, can be short and therefore very time efficient. Benefits can be derived in only a few minutes a day. One of the research studies described above showed positive results with only 20 minutes five times weekly while the other produced results with 5 to 15-minute sessions twice a day.

Convenience: This is one of the most convenient therapies listed in this book. Unless your child used a provider, he or she can use the training material almost anywhere and practice this technique literally anywhere and at any time that it is appropriate to do so.

Other: Another beneficial aspect of meditation is that it has been shown to be helpful for other conditions associated with ADHD, such as anxiety. Also, you as the parent can easily learn this technique using the same material as your child. This will not only help you to be a good role model, but it can be of great benefit in helping you to reduce the stress in your life.

Recommended reading and websites:

www.learningmeditation.com

www.meditationcenter.com
www.meditationsociety.com

Meditating with Children–The Art of Concentration and Centering: A Workbook on New Educational Methods Using Meditation
Author: Deborah Rozman
Integral Yoga Publications Copyright 2002

Teaching Meditation to Children: A Practical Guide to the Use and Benefits of Meditation Techniques
Authors: David Fontana & Ingrid Slack
Element Books Copyright 1998

Contact information:

There is no specific contact information since there are many sources for this information. The books and websites listed above should help you in obtaining the information you need.

Yoga

Names:

Yoga
Hatha Yoga

What it is:

Yoga is a system of exercises that encourages the union of the body, the mind, and the spirit. In fact, the word yoga is derived from a Sanskrit word meaning "to join or yoke together." There is evidence that yoga was practiced as early as 5,000 years ago.

The goal of yoga is to achieve balance and harmony between the mind and body. Some of its benefits include the following:

- increased flexibility and stamina

- stronger muscles

- improved balance and concentration
- improved circulation
- reduced stress and anxiety

Currently, several different styles or types of yoga are being taught and practiced. Each type has its own practices and philosophies. While some yoga styles are meditative and focused on spiritual centeredness, other styles of yoga are more physical and based on physical postures, called poses or asanas. Hatha yoga, which is a system of physical exercises, breathing, relaxation techniques, and meditation, is most often followed by Western yoga practitioners today.[5]

If a class is described as Hatha style, it will likely be slow-paced and gentle or with a flow from one pose to another for aerobic benefits. Beginner classes of Hatha yoga can provide a good introduction to the basic yoga poses. The postures, or poses, include standing, balancing, forward extensions, backward extensions, inversions, and twists. One of the most common poses is "downward facing dog" called Adho Mukha Svanasana. It may likely be the first yoga pose encountered as one begins a yoga practice. It is a transitional pose, a resting pose, and a strengthening pose.

In addition to practicing the poses, yoga classes may also include instruction on relaxation techniques, breathing, meditation, call and response chanting, or an inspirational reading by the teacher. The amount and variety of these components will depend on the instructors and the particular tradition in which they have been trained.

Generally, a yoga class at a gym will be more focused on the purely physical benefits of yoga, while one conducted at a yoga center may delve more into the spiritual side. Some people find that the physical practice of yoga leads them into a more spiritual exploration while others simply enjoy a low-impact workout which makes them feel great.

How it works:

Yoga aims for the perfect union of body, mind, and spirit. It concentrates on the following areas: (1) postures, (2) breathing, and (3) meditation. Practicing the various yoga postures produces a number of positive effects. These include strengthening the body, increasing flexibility, encouraging relaxation, improving posture, and increasing circulation. The controlled breathing helps to focus the mind and is important for relaxation and meditation. The deep, slow breathing patterns have a beneficial effect on the respiratory system. The meditative aspect of yoga is beneficial in calming and focusing the mind. All three areas build on and complement each other.

When practiced regularly, yoga offers numerous health benefits. However, the greater benefits of yoga may arguably be the psychological ones. Yoga combines physical activity with self-awareness, which promotes a mind-body connection which many individuals with ADHD lack.

In practicing yoga, individuals are taught deep breathing and relaxation techniques that help center the mind in the present moment. Practitioners are also guided into holding different postures or poses. Each pose is held for an extended time period, as practitioners focus on holding the best posture they can, while breathing calmly and deeply. The postures or poses promote stretching, strengthening, and balancing as the deep breathing promotes relaxation and mental awareness.

Although yoga can be learned from books or videotapes and lends itself to practice at home, beginners initially would be better served by taking classes with a trained yoga teacher. A trained teacher can assist in learning proper breathing and meditation techniques as well as specific postures. In addition, a good teacher can help address any particular needs or physical limitations.

Yoga classes are frequently longer than other exercise classes, typically lasting between 60 and 90 minutes. A yoga class usually begins with a period of quiet. Next, the instructor will take the class through some gentle warm-up exercises progressing into a series of postures, which are each held anywhere from a few seconds to several minutes. Many of the poses have simple names derived from nature or myths and legends, such as the Cat, the Plank, and the Warrior. As the students' abilities improve, they will be taught progressively more difficult poses.

Proper breathing, through the nostrils, is emphasized throughout a yoga class. The instructor may suggest focusing on exhaling during certain postures while inhaling during other poses. Generally, a class will end with a period of deep relaxation with students lying comfortably on the floor in the "corpse pose" also called the Savasana.

Whether attending classes or practicing yoga at home, it is important to exercise in a warm, quiet room. Loose, comfortable clothing is recommended to provide ease of movement. It is also recommended that yoga be practiced barefoot. A special "sticky mat" is often provided in yoga classes to help prevent slipping. Towels, blankets, wooden blocks, belts, and chairs are often used as props to ensure proper alignment.

There appear to be no hard and fast rules concerning how often or when to do yoga. Many instructors, however, recommend a daily routine of 20 to 30 minutes. To be most comfortable, it is best to practice on an empty stomach. While many individuals prefer practicing yoga first thing in the morning when they awake, others find doing yoga before bedtime helps them to fall asleep.

Sessions:

Usually yoga classes last from 60 to 90 minutes. Beginners typically take one or two classes weekly.

Providers:

Most health clubs, YMCAs, YWCAs, and community centers offer yoga classes. Asking friends for references may be a possibility. Another suggestion for finding a local provider would be to go to YogaFinder™ (www.yogafinder.com) on the Internet. One of its links allows you to find yoga classes by country, state, and zip code.

Since yoga instructors are not medical professionals, no licensing is required. However, certification can be obtained through some yoga schools. It is wise to look for an instructor who has several years of experience and who continues to actively study and practice yoga.

Cost:

As with most other therapies discussed in this book, the cost of yoga classes may vary considerably depending upon the area of the country and who is providing the service. However, you might expect to pay somewhere around $10 to $25 per class.

A number of yoga centers allow new students to take a first class for free. Others periodically offer a complementary shorter version of a regular yoga class for prospective students. While classes are recommended for beginners, there are also many yoga books and videotapes available to guide you.

Research:
Yoga vs. Cooperative Activities

One study conducted in Australia investigated the effects of a yoga practice program on the attention and behavior of 14 boys, ages 8 to 13.[6] All of the boys were diagnosed according to DSM-IV criteria by experienced pediatricians specializing in ADHD. All subjects were randomly assigned to either a yoga group or a control (cooperative activities) group. Although all but two of the boys were stabilized on medication, they were generally not medicated outside of school hours.

Before and after assessments included the Conners' Parent and Teacher Rating Scales-Revised, the Test of Variables of Attention (TOVA), and the motion logger actigraph. The actigraph is a portable electronic activity monitor designed to be worn on the wrist, waist, or ankle. For this study, its purpose was to track the subjects' movements in a number of natural settings, such as at school, at home, and on the weekends, in order to gauge any differences between settings and differences while on and off medication. The actigraph was worn for four consecutive days, two of which were on the weekend.

Twenty weekly one-hour yoga group sessions were conducted at a local medical facility outside of school hours. In addition, parents of the yoga group participants were encouraged to assist with daily practice sessions at home. Participants in the control group engaged in cooperative games and activities that involved the following skills: listening, turn-taking, sharing equipment, and talk time. These activities were conducted once a month for one hour at the same location as the yoga group sessions.

The yoga sessions included practice in respiratory training, postural training, relaxation training, and concentration training. The intent of the respiratory training was to increase the child's breath awareness as well as to train him to breathe naturally through both the mouth and nose. All exercises were repeated several times during each session. The postural training included stretching, backward and forward bends, extensions and inversions performed in sitting, standing, lying face up, and lying face down. The relaxation training focused on becoming progressively more aware of and relaxing body parts and tensing and relaxing muscles. During the concentration training component, a technique called Trataka was used. Using this technique the boys began by mentally focusing on a word or shape. This was followed by the boys seeing the image with their eyes closed and continuing to visualize the image on a blank piece of paper.

Attendance at the yoga classes ranged from 5 to 19 sessions, with 13 (out of 20) being the average number of sessions attended. The number of practice sessions (completed at home) ranged from 14 to 116, with an average of 54.

Comparison of the parental rating scale before and after treatment indicated both the yoga and the control groups showed positive results in several areas. Improvements were found on eight subscales for the yoga group: Oppositional, Global Index Emotional Reactivity, Global Index Total, Global Index Restless/Impulsive, ADHD Index, Perfectionism, DSM-IV Hyperactive/Impulsive, and DSM-IV Total. The control group improved on six subscales: Hyperactivity, Anxious/Shy, Social Problems, Perfectionism, DSM-IV Hyperactive/Impulsive, and DSM-IV Total. In contrast, no significant improvements were indicated in the post-treatment assessment completed by the boys' teachers for either the yoga or control group.

Results:

This particular study on the effects of yoga as a potential complementary ADHD treatment was reviewed in the July 2004 issue of *Attention Research Update*. The results were described as inconclusive, due to a number of factors.

The first concern identified was the small number of participants. We are reminded that even when significant results are obtained, findings which are based on a small and non-representative sample should only be considered as preliminary. The study definitely needs to be replicated with a larger group of participants.[7]

Another concern listed was that while the boys in the yoga group improved in several areas according to the parental rating scale, the participants in the control group also improved in a number of areas. Although the two groups were not compared directly, there was little evidence to indicate that yoga was any more helpful than the supervised, cooperative group activity (control group).

A third concern was that the teacher ratings did not show any significant improvement after the yoga intervention. Indeed, the limitation of the teachers only observing the boys during school hours while they were under medication was brought up by the authors in the discussion section of the article itself. As a result, the authors suggested that any improvement in behavior would be more difficult for the teachers to observe. While this viewpoint is understandable, the results of the study do not provide any indication that yoga training can enhance the functioning of children with ADHD at school. Whether any improved behaviors would have been observed if the boys had not been treated with medication remains unknown.

Pros & cons:

Cautions: The effects of yoga on ADHD are inconclusive at this time. Ensuring that a qualified instructor is going to be providing this training is very important, as some of the positions may be harmful if not performed correctly.

Time: Yoga can be time consuming when considering the length of the sessions as well as the number of sessions that may be required.

Convenience: Since the classes are usually provided at a yoga studio, you will need to find a provider who is conveniently located to you. While yoga is offered in most parts of the country, the locations where it is offered would not be considered numerous. However, once an individual learns the basics, it can be easily done in your home, with or without the aid of books or video tapes.

Other: One of the really beneficial aspects of yoga is that many forms are suitable for almost everyone. The discipline is practiced by people of all ages.

Recommended reading and websites:

www.yogafinder.com
www.yoga.about.com

Complete Idiot's Guide to Yoga with Kids
Authors: Jodi Komitor & Eve Adamson
Alpha Copyright 2000

Contact information:

There is no specific contact information as yoga providers are independent of any central company or organization. However, finding a provider should be fairly easy as most are listed in the phone book. You might also check the local health clubs, YMCAs, YWCAs, and community centers. The website listed above is another source for contacting a provider.

10

Physical Exercise

* Aerobic Exercise

* Tai Chi

Until fairly recently experts believed that new brain cells could not be generated, that the brain cells an individual had at birth had to last for a lifetime. Research in the last few years has shown that the brain has much more plasticity. It is like a muscle; it grows when it is used. Brain cells are created, grow and link to other cells in response to being used. Exercise promotes this brain growth.

The fact that physical exercise is good for the mind and the brain has been known for decades. It is an excellent treatment for ADHD, depression, anxiety, and many other conditions. Regular exercise acts as an antidepressant and an anti-anxiety agent. Psychiatry, however, has tended to separate physical exercise from mainstream treatments.[1]

Physical exercise fuels the production of epinephrine, dopamine, and serotonin, which is exactly what the various medications used to treat ADHD do. Exercising, therefore, is like taking medication for ADHD in a natural, holistic way. Exercise also triggers the release of a brain-derived neurotropic factor (BDNF). This factor enhances cognition by boosting the ability of neurons to communicate with one another. BDNF is important in stimulating the growth of new neurons.[2] Therefore, pursuing a physical (or an intellectual) activity stimulates the growth of new brain cells.

In this chapter we will look at different types of exercise which have been shown to help ADHD. In addition we have included some suggestions and

118

other ideas to consider in implementing an exercise program with your ADHD child.

Aerobic Exercise

Names:

Aerobic Exercise
Cardiovascular Exercise

What it is:

The American College of Sports Medicine defines aerobic exercise as "any activity that uses large muscle groups, can be maintained continuously, and is rhythmic in nature." There are numerous types of aerobic exercise. Among them are walking, running, jogging, jumping rope, stair climbing, swimming, rowing, aerobic dance, and cross country skiing.

How it works:

Aerobic means "with oxygen" and aerobic exercise increases blood circulation and the oxygen and glucose that reach the brain. Movement and exercise increase breathing and heart rate so that more blood flows to the brain, enhancing energy production and waste removal.

Dopamine, a neurotransmitter naturally produced in the brain, plays a key role in modifying mental and physical activity. Dopamine insufficiency can result in a wide range of difficulties, including loss of motor control, poor memory, attention deficit, and depression. It is believed that medications used to treat ADHD increase the amount of chemicals such as dopamine available for work within the brain, especially in the frontal area.[3]

During aerobic exercise, you repeatedly move large muscles in your arms, legs, and hips. In addition to taking in more oxygen, and pumping blood faster and more forcefully, regular aerobic exercise releases endorphins. This release of endorphins during continuous exercise results in a sense of euphoria that has been popularly labeled in recent years as "runner's high." Endorphins are actually good for health and are believed to produce four key effects on the body/mind connection: they (1) enhance the immune system, (2) relieve pain, (3) reduce stress, and (4) postpone the aging process.[4]

Sessions:

Exercising 30 to 45 minutes at least five times a week would be optimal. A warm-up and cool-down (with stretching) period of 5 to 10 minutes at each session is very important as well.

The exercise should be performed at 60 to 75% of maximal heart rate. Maximal heart rate is estimated as 220 minus your age. Heart rate can be calculated by counting your pulse for 15 seconds and multiplying the beats by four. You can teach this technique to your child.

At the beginning of an exercise program, it is advisable to aim for the lower target heart rate (60%). As your fitness level improves, you can exercise harder to get the heart rate closer to the higher number (75%).

Providers:

There are many types of exercise facilities that offer a variety of aerobic exercise classes. Attending exercise classes may provide more motivation for some individuals. However, it is not necessary to attend a class as aerobic exercises can easily be done at home.

Cost:

The price of joining an exercise facility varies greatly. Family plans are generally available with costs ranging from $20 to $100 monthly. There is typically an initial joining fee as well as a contract of six months or more.

However, if you choose to do your exercises at home, in most cases the cost is minimal. Investing, however, in some equipment may be necessary, such as a good pair of running/walking shoes, cross country skis, or a jump rope.

Research:
Classroom Study Using Jogging

Students (12 boys) from first through sixth grade displaying both behavioral and/or perceptual disorders were involved in a morning jog as part of their regular school day over a six-week period.[5] Both a warm-up and cool-down period were a part of each jogging routine. The jogging period, from warm-up to the beginning of class work, was approximately 15 minutes. The teacher of this self-contained classroom jogged regularly with her students. On some days, students were allowed to simply exercise during this period if they had medical excuses, colds, or a note from home.

The teacher established a random three times a week schedule during which the day and the amount of time spent jogging varied. Each Monday, Wednesday, and Friday of the six-week period the children spent either five, ten, or no minutes jogging.

Five types of negative behaviors (hitting/bothering others, name calling/throwing things, yelling/talking out of turn, moving or sitting inappropriately, refusing to cooperate or participate) were identified by the classroom teacher prior to the beginning of the study. The number of incidents of each of the negative behaviors was recorded for each time block each day of the study, and the results were combined for a daily total. A comparison of the negative behaviors occurring on jogging versus non-jogging days showed that disruptive behaviors on jogging days were reduced by 50%. The average number of negative behaviors observed on jogging days was 32 (for ten minutes of jogging) and 37 (for five minutes of jogging). In contrast, on the days with no jogging the average number of daily classroom disruptions was 63.

The fewest disruptive behaviors occurred in the first hour immediately following the jogging. In comparison, on the days when the children did not jog, the first hour of class had twice as many disruptions. Additionally, the teacher's informal observations indicated that on days when the children jogged, they seemed better able to attend to their academic tasks. They also displayed a more positive attitude toward school.

Intense Aerobic Summer Activity Program

Children diagnosed with ADHD participated in intense aerobic activity for six weeks during the summer.[6] Medicated and non-medicated children, ranging in age from 5 to 12, were accepted for the study. There were 13 participants (12 boys and 1 girl) in the exercise group and 11 participants (9 boys and 2 girls) in the control group.

The exercise sessions occurred five times a week (Monday through Friday) for 40 minutes. Each child's respiration rate was monitored throughout the activity period. The Polar Heart Rate Monitor, an electronic device that can measure and store an individual's heart rate history, was used with each participant. The researcher programmed all of the monitors for the participants prior to the first exercise session. The monitors were programmed for 10 minutes of warm-up, 20 minutes of intense exercise, and 10 minutes of cool-down. Since the monitors provided a constant reading for average heart rate, the researcher was able to adjust the exercise sessions for each child based on the monitor's output.

If a participant was not reaching the pre-designed zone, efforts were made to motivate the child to the desired level of exercise intensity, which was 75 percent of maximum heart rate. As the program progressed over the six-week time frame, the need to motivate the children into the zone grew less. According to the researcher, they seemed empowered to reach the zone on their own initiative.

Age-specific activities were used to maintain each individual's interest during the daily exercise sessions. Running, aerobic games, video fitness, exercise stations, tag games, and jump rope activities were some of the exercises used.

Using the Conners' Short Form Parent Rating Scale (CPRS), behavior profiles were given to both the parents of the exercise group and the parents of the control group just prior to the beginning of the exercise session and just after the last day of the program. Results from the pre-treatment CPRS profile showed both groups to be "Markedly Atypical/Moderately Atypical" which indicates a significant problem.

Results from the post treatment profile showed that the exercise group had improved. The profile showed the exercise group to be "Average/Mildly Atypical," which only indicates a possible problem. Conversely, the control group profile showed no change.

Significant positive changes occurred for the exercise group in four specific areas of the Conners' rating scale: oppositional index, hyperactivity index, inattention index, and cognitive problems. Looking at the post-assessment data from the Conners' Parent Rating Form, the control group showed no significant changes in their behavior.

Parents' comments on the post-program evaluation form included various positive responses regarding their child's behavior and participation in the summer activity program. Children were described as "less argumentative and more cooperative," "less aggressive and more focused," "more manageable and much calmer," and "not bouncing all over and more pleasant."

Running Study Described in Running as Therapy: An Integrated Approach

In this study running group participants were involved in slow long-distance running sessions for 45 minutes four times weekly for 12 weeks.[7] Six weeks of training preceded the 12 weeks of the study. A total of 56 ADHD children, ranging in age from 6 to 13, participated. Each running group averaged eight children, with two adult staff members as leaders. The running group leaders recorded the amount each group member ran.

While improvements is aggression, impulsivity, and hyperactivity were observed, the most notable finding, according to the researcher, was that running made it possible to reduce psycho-stimulant medication dosages. Although doctors did not know which children were involved in the running treatment and which ones were not, stimulant dosages for a sizeable number of children in the running group were reduced. As a rule, the more a child ran, the less medication was required. After the study, children who stopped running reverted to their previous behaviors.

Results:

The results of the studies above are quite promising. While the time it took to initially see the improvements is not clear, it is obvious that results were identified within a six-week period. There also appears to be a correlation between the amount of exercise and level of improvements with one study showing that the more the child ran, the less medication was needed. However, the benefits appear to be relatively short-lived as most of the improvements tapered off if the exercise was not continued.

Pros & cons:

Cautions: As with any exercise plan, you should make sure that your child has no medical conditions that would cause concern before starting an aerobic exercise plan.

Time: The amount of time it takes to produce positive results is surprisingly minimal. In one of the studies, a 50% reduction in disruptive behaviors was achieved in exercising as little as 15 minutes only three days a week. However, those results declined rapidly and were non-existent on the days that the children did not run. For longer lasting results, it appears your child would need to continue to maintain a regular program of exercise.

Convenience: If your child is motivated, doing aerobic exercises is very convenient. Just find something that he or she likes to do that is aerobic and turn him or her loose. It is also very convenient if your child's school provides this type of exercise as part of their physical education program. However, if your child is addicted to the high stimulus of video games, you may need to make a real effort at engaging in an aerobic activity with him or her. This is where a health club may be worth the time and money. It may appear less suitable to choose this option, but in reality it may prove to be well worth it.

Other: Suggestions and Ideas
Physical Exercise Suggestions from The ADD Answer

According to Dr. Lawlis, while all children benefit from regular physical exercise, those with ADHD particularly need to be physically active to keep the blood flowing to their brains. He recommends three exercises to teachers for use before each class to enhance attention span and focus. These are: (1) relaxation therapies such as deep breathing, (2) muscle stretching exercises, and (3) toning exercises.[8]

During the first or relaxation phase, students are instructed to make themselves comfortable. They are told to focus on an object or particular space on the wall. This stage lasts about three minutes, and the idea is to have the children focus their energy on their beating hearts.

In the second or muscle stretching phase, attention is given to the muscles of the arms, legs, and back. Although the exact exercises appear not to be critical, the exercise involving a flower awakening is described by the author. The initial position has the children curled up on the floor, with them slowly stretching out their arms and neck as if they were flowers growing from the floor and reaching skyward for rain or sunshine. There are no set procedures or rules for bending and stretching. However, at the end the children are standing with their arms and legs extended. This second stage should also last about three minutes.

The third or final phase is the toning exercise. During this stage the children are asked to hum a tone, or perhaps a song, that stimulates or wakes up the brain for about two to three minutes. The idea is for them to find a tone that causes vibrations in their heads. With a whole group of children, the classroom may become quite loud. As long as the children are concentrating on their empowerment and their breathing, the extra noise should not be a concern.

Comment: Although this is described for a classroom of children, we don't see why you as a parent might not want to try this strategy at home. With only you and your child, the room won't be as noisy. Joining your child in doing this exercise should enhance the experience. You may also want to share this technique with your child's teacher.

Tips in Choosing Sports for Your ADHD Child from The A.D.D. Book

Since sports can be either a positive or a negative experience for the ADHD child, parents need some suggestions for matching their child to an appropriate sport.[9] Some factors to think about are as follows:

- Consider your child's temperament and set him or her up for success.

- If group situations are difficult for your child, consider getting semiprivate or private lessons first, until your child feels more confident. Confidence is very important in helping your child to settle down long enough to cooperate in group instruction.

- Know your child. If your child enjoys more action, he or she will probably be better off playing soccer than baseball.

- Don't be in a hurry to invest in equipment. Wait until you feel confident your child will stick with the sport.

- Practice with your child. Generally children will maintain interest if they have more skills before they join a team. Therefore, spending time in the weeks prior to the start of official practice can pay big dividends. Children who are more confident in their abilities and experience success are much more likely to stick with a sport.

- Match your child with the right position on the team. For example, in Little League baseball, an infield position is much better for an ADHD child than the outfield. More action is happening in the infield. Being the pitcher or catcher may be the appropriate spot. Remember that intense focus can give an athlete with ADHD an edge, so think about your child being in the center of the action.

- Consider martial arts for your child. Sports like karate, or Tai Chi which is a form of karate, can be therapeutic since they allow a child to be aggressive in a controlled way. They require the individual to stand in a certain spot and listen to instructions. Indeed, your child may be more attentive because the instructions make sense and have immediate relevance. (p. 162)

Recommended reading and websites:

Nature's Ritalin for the Marathon Mind: Nurturing Your ADHD Child with Exercise
Author: Stephen C. Putnam
Upper Access, Inc., Book Publishers Copyright 2001

Delivered from Distraction: Getting the Most out of Life with Attention Deficit Disorder
Author: Edward M. Hallowell, M.D. & John J. Ratey, M.D.
Ballantine Books Copyright 2005

Chapter 8 "Emotional and Behavioral Effects of Long-Distance Running on Children" by Shipman, W. M. found in *Running as Therapy: An Integrated Approach* by M.L. Sachs & G.W. Buffone (Eds.) (1985).

Contact information:

Using your local phone book may be the best way to find a health club in your area.

Tai Chi

Names:

Tai Chi (pronounced "tie chee")
Tai Chi Chuan

What it is:

Tai Chi is a gentle exercise routine which is part of Traditional Chinese Medicine. It can perhaps best be thought of as a moving form of yoga and meditation combined. There are a number of forms, which are sometimes referred to as "sets," that consist of a sequence of movements.

Many of these movements, which were originally derived from the martial arts, incorporate natural movements of birds and animals. In Tai Chi, these movements are performed slowly, deliberately, and gracefully with smooth and even transitions between them.

Although Tai Chi has been practiced in China for centuries and is still a daily regimen for millions of people in the East, it first came to the United States in the early 1970s. Since its introduction, Tai Chi has grown in popularity among all age groups. It is designed to enhance overall health through (1) meditation, (2) slow, graceful movements, and (3) deep breathing.

How it works:

Tai Chi is based on spiritual and philosophical ideas that advocate a need for balance in the human mind, body, and spirit. Central to Tai Chi is the concept that a life force, or Qi (pronounced "chee"), flows throughout the body by means of channels called meridians. When this life force flows properly, the mind, body, and spirit are in balance and good health is maintained. The Qi also depends on the balance of the two opposing energies of Yin and Yang. Yin and Yang are opposite and complementary forces in nature, such as light/dark or feminine/masculine. It is believed that performing Tai Chi serves to harmonize these two energy forces and therefore enhances the balance of the mind, body, and spirit.

There is more than one perspective on how Tai Chi works. As described in the previous paragraph, Eastern philosophy holds that Tai Chi unblocks the flow of Qi and when Qi flows properly, the mind, body, and spirit are balanced and health is maintained. Another view is that Tai Chi works in much the same way as other mind/body therapies. This view is supported by the existing evidence that the connection between the mind and the body can be used to relieve stress, combat disease, and enhance both mental and physical well-being.

There are various benefits derived from regularly practicing the three main components of Tai Chi: movement, meditation, and deep breathing. Since all the major muscle groups and joints are needed to perform the slow and graceful movements, this gentle exercise program improves balance, agility, strength, flexibility, stamina, muscle tone, and coordination. In addition, the beneficial aspects of meditation include improving concentration, reducing anxiety, and lowering blood pressure and heart rate. Finally, deep breathing increases lung capacity, stretches the muscles involved in breathing, releases tension, and improves blood circulation to the brain, thus boosting mental alertness.

Sessions:

Tai Chi sessions are usually group classes which last about an hour. A session begins with a warm-up exercise. This is followed by the instructor guiding the class through a series of forms, each made up of a succession of movements. Each form has a nature-based name that describes its overall action, such as "grasp the bird's tail" or "wave hands like clouds." All movements are to be performed in a slow, meditative manner while focusing on breathing deeply. At the end of each session there is a cool-down, relaxation, and meditation time.

Most instructors will probably recommend practicing Tai Chi daily at home since regular practice is essential for mastering the forms and achieving lasting results. It will take time to develop the agility and flexibility needed for Tai Chi.

Because Tai Chi exercises all the major muscle groups in the body, it is not unusual to feel sore when first beginning a Tai Chi program.

Providers:

For information on finding a Tai Chi class in your area, you might begin by contacting local health clubs or perhaps the YMCA or YWCA. Health food stores and the local newspaper may also have ads about these classes. There are also various websites on the Internet that have links to a variety of Tai Chi sites and organizations which may be of assistance in finding an instructor or class. See recommended Internet websites listed at the end of the chapter.

Cost:

Since there is no special equipment to buy and use, the cost of this treatment option is quite minimal. The only cost involved will be the weekly Tai Chi lessons. Insurance would generally not cover these classes, as they would be considered just another exercise.

The cost for Tai Chi varies depending upon the area or region of the country in which the classes are provided as well as who teaches the classes. The price of group classes will probably range from $10 to $25 per class but monthly or package discounts are often available. Individual lessons are usually available for an additional fee.

Research:
Effects of Tai Chi on ADHD

One study examined the effects of Tai Chi on anxiety, mood, hyperactivity, and conduct in children with ADHD.[10] Eleven boys and two girls, ranging in age from 13 to 16, participated in Tai Chi classes twice a week for five weeks.

Each Tai Chi class was 30 minutes in length and occurred during the middle of the afternoon. All ten sessions began with the students slowly raising and lowering their arms in synchrony with breathing exercises for a five-minute period. In addition, the children were taught to perform slow turning and twisting movements of the arms and legs, shifting their body weight from one leg to the other, rotating from side to side, and changing directions in a sequence of Tai Chi forms.

The Conners' Teacher Rating Scale was used to determine the effectiveness of the Tai Chi lessons. This 28-item assessment instrument has a total hyperactivity score as well as scores in the following subcategories: (1) anxiety, (2) asocial behavior, (3) conduct, (4) daydreaming, (5) emotion, and (6) hyperactivity.

Teachers completed this rating scale at three separate times for the study. The first time was two weeks before the participants began Tai Chi classes for a baseline assessment. The second time was at the end of the five-week Tai Chi program to measure the effect of the classes. The third, and final time, was two weeks after the last class had been conducted to measure the carry-over effect or benefit of Tai Chi.

After taking Tai Chi for the five-week period, the children displayed less anxiety, improved conduct, less daydreaming, less inappropriate emotions, and less hyperactivity. It is very important to note that these improved behaviors, as observed by their teachers, continued over the two week follow-up period when the children no longer were taking Tai Chi.

Although this appears to be the only pediatric study involving ADHD children and Tai Chi, there are adult and geriatric studies reporting the benefits of Tai Chi in reducing symptoms associated with stress and stress hormone levels. These same studies identify its positive effect on mood and psychosocial well-being.

Results:

The results for Tai Chi and ADHD are very promising. As stated above, in just 10 sessions done only twice a week for 30 minutes, positive results were noted. Compared to aerobic exercises, the benefits of doing Tai Chi appear to be sustained over a longer period of time. If your child were to do the exercises on a daily basis, it may be possible that the results would be more pronounced with even more carry-over.

Pros & cons:

Cautions: Even though Tai Chi is considered to be a safe and effective form of exercise and relaxation for almost everyone, it is not meant to replace medical care. Therefore, it is always wise to consult your child's physician and the Tai Chi instructor before beginning this or any other exercise program.

Time: The time commitment will include a weekly class of about an hour as well as daily practices at home. One source we found indicated that many instructors recommend practicing for about 15 to 20 minutes twice daily between classes. However, visiting with your Tai Chi instructor will help you determine this, along with your child's interest.

Convenience: It will be necessary to find a Tai Chi class offered at a time that works with your child's other regularly scheduled activities, such as school, homework, etc. Obviously, there is considerable flexibility as to when the daily practices at home could be completed. If the classes become too inconvenient after your child had achieved the basics of Tai Chi, a video can be purchased that would allow him/her to continue the exercises at home using the training video.

Other: One of the advantages of this treatment is that the parents or even the whole family would generally benefit from doing Tai Chi along with the child. This would not only encourage the child to do the exercise, but the benefits to a family under stress could be substantial.

Recommended reading and websites:

www.holisticmed.com/www/qigong.html—Tai Chi Internet Resources
www.mtsu.edu/~jpurcell/Taichi/tc-links.htm—Tai Chi Internet links
usataichi.org—The USA National Tai Chi Chuan Federation
www.taichinetwork.org—Tai Chi Network
www.taichinetwork.org/list_search.cfm—Tai Chi Network search for classes
www.tai-chi.com/magazine.htm *T'AI CHI* Magazine

T'AI CHI Magazine
Wayfarer Publications
P.O. Box 39938
Los Angeles, CA 90039
Phone: USA (800) 888-9119

Contact information:

The USA National Tai Chi Chuan Federation
991 Main Street
Manchester, Connecticut 06040
Phone: (860) 646-6818
E-mail: info@usataichi.org

Tai Chi Network—Phone: (603) 227-9185
Information on Tai Chi classes in your area

11

Homeopathy

Names:

Homeopathy
Homeopathics
Homeopathic Medicine
Homeotherapeutics

What it is:

Homeopathy, the second most widely used system of medicine in the world, is an alternative, natural, complementary medicine based on the Law of Similars, minimal dose, and the single remedy. The "Law of Similars" (like cures like) holds that the same substance which causes disease in healthy people can cure the disease in someone who is ill. A German physician named Samuel Hahnemann, who is known as the founder of homeopathy, is said to have based his theory on an experience in which he swallowed cinchona bark, the source of quinine which is used to treat malaria. After eating the bark, Dr. Hahnemann experienced thirst, throbbing in the head, and fever. All of these are symptoms common to malaria. Consequently, he decided that the drug's power to cure the disease arose from its ability to produce symptoms similar to the disease itself.

The "Principle of Minimum Dose" is based on the idea that extreme dilution enhances the curative properties of a substance while eliminating any possible side effects. Dr. Hahnemann created small doses by repeatedly diluting the original substance in a mixture of water and alcohol until it was no longer toxic.

Homeopathic physicians often use medicines made with 30, 200, 1,000, or 10,000 dilutions, which far exceed the point at which molecules of the original substance remain in the solution. This seems impossible and no one really understands how the information pattern in homeopathic remedies persists during dilution beyond the disappearance of the physical molecules of the original substance.

Homeopathy is practiced throughout the world, including Europe, India, Pakistan, South Africa, and South America. Nearly 50% of British physicians refer to homeopaths and other practitioners of complementary medicine. Homeopathic medicines are available in over 20,000 pharmacies in France, and approximately 40% of French physicians have prescribed the medicines. In India, there are more than 120 homeopathic medical schools and approximately 100,000 homeopaths.

Homeopathic medicines come from all over the world. Indeed, virtually any naturally occurring substance can be utilized as a homeopathic remedy. Medicines are made from the animal, plant, and mineral kingdoms. A few of the homeopathic medicines which have been used successfully in treating ADHD include: Tarentula hispanica (secreted by the tarantula spider), Veratrum album (white hellebore), Stramonium (datura stramonium), Belladonna (deadly nightshade), Arsenicum iodatum (iodide of arsenic), Zincum metallicum (zinc), and Argentum nitricum (silver nitrate).[1]

The Food and Drug Administration (FDA) is responsible for regulating homeopathic medicines in the United States. Homeopathic pharmacies are required to follow rigid guidelines established by the Homeopathic Pharmacopoeia of the United States. While some homeopathic medicines are available over the counter in pharmacies or health food stores, others can only be obtained through licensed medical practitioners.

The homeopathic medicines found in most health food stores are called "combination medicines" or "formulas," since they are mixtures of between three to eight different homeopathic medicines. Various manufacturers select the medicines most commonly prescribed for specific symptoms and assume that one of them will help cure the ailment the consumer has. These "user friendly" combination medicines are quite popular in the United States and Europe because they are so easy to prescribe and because they tend to be effective. However, combination medicines found over the counter would not be preferred for conditions such as ADHD. While these medicines are valuable, most professional homeopaths have found that the medicine individually chosen for the person tends to work more often and more deeply.

How it works:

As described above, homeopathy is based on the "Law of Similars." This basically means that like cures like. In other words, the same substance which causes disease in healthy people can cure the disease in someone who is ill. Simply put, homeopathy takes an extremely diluted form of a substance that will produce the same symptoms as the disease which one wants to cure and gives it to the patient. Contrary to what one would expect, this substance causes the body to respond in such a way as to cure the disorder rather than making it worse.

While conventional medical doctors often treat a patient's condition with various kinds of drugs, a homeopathic focus is on treating the whole person, rather than the disease. A homeopathic practitioner also uses only a single medicine at a time which is individualized according to the patient's unique pattern of symptoms. This is determined by taking a complete, detailed patient history. These medicines are used to heal physical as well as mental and emotional symptoms including those of ADHD. Homeopathy uses natural, nontoxic medicines that typically last for months or years, rather than hours.

There is only one homeopathic medicine at any point in time that will have the most impact on an individual's condition. A trained and experienced homeopathic practitioner's job is to find that one specific medicine that most closely matches the patient's symptoms. When the match is made well and the prescription is correct, the patient's condition will noticeably improve. Therefore, each patient with ADHD may need a different homeopathic remedy.

Homeopathic medicines are available in pill or in liquid form. The specific way of taking the medication depends upon the medicine itself, its potency, the condition being treated, and the sensitivity of the patient. A few drops of liquid or a few pills may be given at one time. However, the exact method and the repetition of medicine depend upon all of the previously mentioned factors.

While there are no lists of potential side effects from particular homeopathic substances, there are certain symptoms an individual may experience as part of the healing process. Some of these include a brief flare-up or aggravation of already existing symptoms within the first week of taking a homeopathic medicine and a brief return of old symptoms. Both the aggravation and the re-experiencing of past symptoms are typically a sign that the medicine is a good match. Generally, these symptoms are followed by a significant improvement. It is rare for an individual to experience a new symptom after taking a homeopathic medicine, but if this does occur, you should check with your homeopath.

Often children are already on Ritalin or other medications when they begin homeopathic treatment. It is common in this situation for children to continue their medication until the homeopath finds the correct medicine for the child. At times, it may take several tries of different homeopathic medicines before the optimal one is found. When the appropriate match has been made and the child's symptoms show considerable improvement, it is strongly recommended that parents consult with their medical physician or pediatrician concerning discontinuing or reducing the conventional medications. It is also extremely important to tell your homeopath what your child is like when off all medications.

Sessions:

There are no sessions as such in using this modality. The homeopathic medication can easily be taken at home. However, it is recommended that you use a homeopathic practitioner for an initial assessment and periodic check-ups to ensure that your child receives the optimal benefits of this treatment.

Your first visit to a homeopathic practitioner will consist of a thorough, detailed evaluation of your child's medical history, behaviors, ADHD symptoms, etc. Other sessions will focus on assessing the effectiveness of the medicines and developing new protocols as needed.

When beginning treatment, visits with your homeopathic practitioner are typically scheduled every six to eight weeks. However, after your child has responded well to treatment, your homeopath may only need to see your child two or three times a year to help maintain optimal health.

Although significant progress is often reported within the first one to three months, it is recommended that most children continue under the care of a homeopath for at least two years. This is something you definitely will want to discuss with your homeopathic physician.

Providers:

Homeopathy is practiced by a wide range of health care providers, including medical doctors, doctors of osteopathy, naturopathic doctors, chiropractors, nurse practitioners, physician assistants, dentists, nurses, acupuncturists, and podiatrists, as well as professional homeopaths. Most homeopaths undergo three or four years of training, which includes specific work in case analysis which allows them to learn the finely developed skills of matching the appropriate remedy to specific symptoms. Most naturopathic colleges have programs in homeopathy. In fact, it is very common for naturopathic doctors (N.D.s) to use homeopathy in their practices. Homeopathic practitioners who attend naturopathic school also fulfill medical school-like training and clinical applications. Many homeopaths are also medical doctors, doctors of osteopathy, chiropractors, and naturopathic doctors.

In selecting a homeopathic practitioner, it is essential to ask whether the practitioner is certified in homeopathy since there are a few individuals who practice homeopathy with very little formal training. According to the National Center for Homeopathy's website (www.homeopathic.org/ find.htm), the Certified Classical Homeopath (CCH) credential is excellent. The Diplomate in Homeotherapeutics (or DHt credential) is available for medical doctors and doctors of osteopathy and the Diplomate of the Homeopathic Academy of Naturopathic Physicians (DHANP) certification is available for naturopathic physicians. Even though there are numerous skilled homeopaths, you may wish to see a medical or naturopathic doctor who practices homeopathy in the case of treating ADHD.

The choices of providers available to use will vary according to where you live. If you reside in a major metropolitan area, you will undoubtedly have more choices, although many practitioners are located throughout the United States.

Cost:

The cost of homeopathic care will vary considerably from one homeopath to another. As a general rule, medical doctors who practice homeopathy will charge more than non-M.D. practitioners. Another factor is experience; the longer homeopaths have been practicing, the higher their fees tend to be.

The initial visit to a homeopath will usually take at least an hour and very possibly more than an hour. If you choose an M.D. homeopath, you will find the fees for this first visit comparable with other physician specialists, so the cost will likely range from $100 to $300. Other homeopaths, who are not medical doctors, will charge anywhere from $50 to $250. Follow-up visits typically cost between $30 and $80 for non-medical doctors, while homeopaths who are also medical doctors may charge from $50 to $100 per visit.

Although medically-trained homeopaths will recommend laboratory tests when indicated, it is rare for them to run such tests to determine the appropriate homeopathic medicine. Therefore, the costs of laboratory tests will likely not be an expense you will need to consider.

Finally, the actual price of the homeopathic medicine itself is insignificant. If only one medicine is prescribed, which is most common, its cost will range between $4.00 and $10.00. It is interesting to note that some homeopaths will provide whatever they prescribe without any charge.

As a general rule, if the type of practitioner is covered by your insurance, such as a medical doctor, doctor of osteopathy, naturopath, or chiropractor, then the visit should be covered. You may want to consider whether the practitioner includes other therapies in his or her practice and if you would wish to use those therapies. As always, your specific coverage questions will need to be addressed to your insurance company.

Research:
A Double Blind, Partial Crossover Study

Forty-three children, diagnosed with ADHD, were alternately assigned to either a placebo or homeopathic treatment group to determine the effectiveness of homeopathy for treating ADHD.[2] All participants (25 boys and 18 girls) were living in foster homes or with their parents under the supervision of social workers. The average age of the children was 10 years. In addition, six of the children were on medications, but all six were still showing signs of ADHD.

In this partial crossover study, after ten days the placebo group was given homeopathics and compared against itself. Since homeopathic medicines are assumed to have lasting effects, it was not possible to do a complete crossover design and switch those initially taking homeopathic medicines to placebos.

A patient history for the selection of homeopathic medicines was obtained at the time of testing. The investigator had no further contact with the children following the initial testing and case-taking interview. The placebo or homeopathic pills were mailed to the parents or caregivers approximately one week following the initial testing. Neither the children nor the individuals administering the pills and rating improvement changes were aware of which pills were the placebos and which were not.

Identical bottles, labeled only with the first name of the child, were used for both the placebos and the homeopathic medicine. Written directions were included explaining how to administer the pills. Six pills were taken daily at one time, for up to five days or until a marked change occurred.

Homeopathic medicines were selected individually for each child based upon his or her unique symptom pattern. Approximately 10 days following each administration of the homeopathic medicines or placebos, the parents and caregivers were contacted by phone to obtain follow-up ratings on behavioral changes.

Parents and caregivers rated changes in hyperactivity according to the following scale: much worse (-2), a little worse (-1), no change (0), a little better (+1), and much better (+2). Changes had to be observed in the home and/or reported by teachers at school. Improvements, when they occurred, were usually reported by about the third day of treatment.

When ratings for children receiving homeopathic remedies indicated little or no improvement, a new medicine was prescribed. A second medicine was given to 18 children and seven of those children required a third medicine. After three tries, no further medicines were administered.

Two behavioral comparisons were conducted. Results in comparing those children who received only one homeopathic medicine to those in the placebo treatment group indicated that the behavior scores or ratings for the homeopathic group were significantly better. In a second comparison, the improvement scores for the children in the placebo group were compared to their scores after they were given homeopathic medicines. These children's scores improved significantly after they were given homeopathics.

Statistically significant differences were found for both comparisons. This finding supports the theory that homeopathic treatment is superior to placebo treatment for ADHD.

Follow-up interviews with the parents and caregivers were conducted approximately two months after the last improvement ratings. Of those children who showed improvement during the study, continued improvement was shown for 57%, without any further use of homeopathic remedies. Although another 24% continued to show improvement for several days or weeks following the taking of the homeopathics, they had relapsed by the time the follow-up interview was conducted. For the remaining 19% of the children, positive results were shown only while they were taking the homeopathic medicines.

Discussion

Stramonium, Cina, and Hyoscyamus niger were the homeopathic medicines identified as most successful in this study. Veratrum album and Tarentula hispanica were also found to be useful, although to a much lesser extent. Since foster mothers were usually responsible for the case history or intake information on each child, it was often the case that the detailed information needed to determine the appropriate medicine was unknown to them. When this information was not available, Stramonium was initially given.

Stramonium was used when the child demonstrated numerous fears or symptoms of post-tramatic stress disorder. It was also indicated when rages of anger occurred in the context of several fears or phobias. Cina was found to be very beneficial for those children who were prone to frequent fighting and arguing and who had tantrums when they were told what to do or disciplined. Hyoscyamus niger was useful with children who displayed any type of sexualized symptom as well as those children who typically exhibited manic sorts of behaviors. Children with which hyoscyamus was most effective were often described as wild or impossible to control. It is important to note that the foster children in this study included many traumatized children, who had been physically and sexually abused.

Comparison of Homeopathy and Traditional Medication in a Family Setting

This Swiss study compared the effectiveness of homeopathy and Ritalin (methylphenidate) for the treatment of ADHD children.[3] Participants (92 boys and 23 girls) ranged in age from 3 to 17 years. An initial assessment of the hyperactivity and attention deficit symptoms according to the Conners' Global Index (CGI) rating scale was conducted on each child prior to the beginning of the study. Children with a CGI score of 14 or higher were included. Additionally, a thorough history was taken prior to each child beginning treatment with homeopathics.

All of the 115 children received an individual homeopathic treatment. The homeopathic medicine was matched to the symptom pattern of each child. Depending on the severity of their symptoms, participants received treatments daily or every second day.

Assessment was based on parental reporting of observed changes in each symptom initially reported on the Conners' 10-item rating scale (CGI). After parents reported the changes in each individual symptom, they were asked to summarize the overall clinical improvement as a percentage. When the overall improvement reached 50% or more, the treatment was reassessed by the CGI rating scale. There was no uniform time when this reassessment occurred. In fact, the timing was completely individualized, depending on the time required to find the correct homeopathic medicine for each child.

Children who did not reach the 50% or higher improvement rating, or whose behavior remained unacceptable despite some response to homeopathy, were changed to the stimulant medication Ritalin (methylphenidate) after being reassessed. Two weeks after stimulant medication treatment was begun, the Conners' Global Index was used to distinguish the responders from the non-responders. The final CGI assessment of the effectiveness of Ritalin occurred three months after the optimal dosage adjustment was determined.

The results of this study showed 75% of the participants (86 children) reached a satisfactory improvement in their behavior using homeopathic medicines. Twenty-five children (or 22%) were changed to stimulant medication while three children (or 3%) did not respond favorably to either treatment. One child left the study. The time needed to reach an optimal homeopathic treatment effect varied from one to 16 months. The average length of homeopathic treatment for those children who were eventually switched to stimulant medication was 22 months, with the range being from four to 62 months.

The observed parental ratings of clinical improvement and the lowering of the CGI under homeopathic treatment were slightly better than under the stimulant medication. Clinical improvement ratings were 73% for the homeopathy-treated children and 65% for stimulant-treated children. A majority of the participants who eventually took stimulant medications had a treatment effect from homeopathy. However, the average clinical improvement for these individuals was 43%, which was substantially lower than in those children who responded favorably to homeopathy.

Discussion

One of the challenges in homeopathy is the time it may take for optimal improvement to be achieved. The homeopathic practitioner selects the appropriate medication by evaluating the individual or unique symptoms of the patient. If the patient only has the "typical" symptoms of ADHD and no unique symptoms, the homeopathic physician may need to make "therapeutic trials" to find the right medication. While choosing the wrong medication is not harmful, making the correct choice leads to a marked improvement within approximately four weeks. In this particular study, the majority of the children who responded favorably to homeopathic treatment did so within six months. If a child has not responded to homeopathy within that time period, it appears unlikely that he or she will.

According to the authors of this study, homeopathy does have several advantages over Ritalin (methylphenidate). First, it is relatively easy to administer, with it being given once daily or once every other day. Secondly, it has a continuous treatment effect which lasts over the entire time period with no rebounding effect. Third, it has basically no side effects, except for a possible short initial aggravation. Last, but certainly not least, homeopathic treatment has no abuse potential.

Results:

The results of the double blind, partial crossover study discussed above indicates that homeopathic treatment is superior to placebo treatment for ADHD. Approximately two months after the last improvement ratings were taken, 57%, of those children who showed improvement during the study, continued to make improvement without any further use of homeopathic remedies. Another 24% continued to show improvement for several days or weeks following the taking of the homeopathics but had relapsed sometime during the two months. For the remaining 19% of the children, positive results were shown only while they were taking the homeopathic medicines.

The results of the second research study on the comparison of homeopathy and traditional medication discussed above showed 75% of the participants reached a satisfactory improvement in their behavior using homeopathic medicines. Twenty-two percent did not make the satisfactory improvements and were changed to stimulant medication to which they did respond favorably while 3% of the children did not respond favorably to either treatment.

In this particular study, the majority of the children who responded favorably to homeopathic treatment did so within six months. If a child has not responded to homeopathy within that time period, it appears unlikely that he or she will.

Expectations of Treatment for ADHD: Taken from Ritalin-Free Kids

According to Drs. Judyth Reichenberg-Ullman and Robert Ullman, a 70% improvement, over time, can be expected in a substantial number of areas for your ADHD child.[4] These areas include: behavior at school and at home, impulsivity, ability to concentrate, ability to make friends, restlessness, mood, grades, self-esteem, appropriate social behavior, physical health complaints, immunity, and overall health.

While these improvements generally begin within two to five weeks after being prescribed the correct homeopathic medicine, they continue and stabilize over time. Because of this, homeopathic treatment is very strongly recommended for at least one to two years. According to these naturopaths, the most profound effects of homeopathy occur when it is continued for a number of years.

Pros & cons:

Cautions: Combination medicines, such as those found in a health food store, should not be used to treat chronic or recurring conditions such as ADHD. (Combination medicines contain a variety of common homeopathic substances which have been found to be beneficial for such conditions as colds or sore throats. If the one medicine needed is contained in that combination, the individual will respond well. However, if it is not, the individual will likely have no response or a partial response to the medicine.) The chances of your child being helped are much greater if you work in conjunction with a trained, experienced homeopathic practitioner. Even then, it may take several tries before finding the right homeopathic remedy.

Certain substances or exposures may interfere with homeopathic treatment, even when the correct remedy has been given. This phenomenon is known as antidoting. Most practitioners will advise you regarding what substances and/ or objects to avoid. Some of the more common ones include: (1) coffee (or anything flavored with coffee, such as ice cream or candy), (2) electric blankets, (3) aromatic substances like camphor, eucalyptus, menthol, and peppermint (some products containing these include Vick's, Noxema, Tiger Balm, Ben Gay, cough drops, toothpaste, mouthwash), and (4) topical medications such as topical steroids, antibiotics, and antifungals. Aromatic lip balms, such as Chapstick and Blistex, should also be avoided. Oral antibiotics and cortisone products should only be used after consulting with your homeopath. In addition, acupuncture, one of the other treatment options described in this book, is not recommended during homeopathic treatment. Homeopathic practitioners may differ in their advice on what to avoid.

Not every person is affected by potentially antidoting substances in the same way. For example, while a sip of coffee is enough to interfere with the process of homeopathic treatment for some individuals, for others it takes a number of exposures before a relapse occurs.

Antidoting may occur at any time, even one or two years after a remedy has been given. When it does occur, symptoms which have been eliminated by homeopathy will likely return. Sometimes the relapse is partial or temporary; at other times the interference is total, causing a sudden, complete relapse. If exposure is suspected, homeopaths generally wait one to two weeks before re-evaluating a case and deciding whether to repeat a patient's remedy. This waiting period is required in order to assess whether the previous symptoms will return and to give the patient an opportunity to bounce back without the need for repeating the remedy.

It is not our intent to worry you in any way by educating you regarding the antidoting phenomenon. By knowing about its existence, you can ask more informed questions of your homeopathic provider. Many homeopaths give their patients a list of which substances to avoid. Other practitioners, however, do not make this phenomenon an issue until or unless it actually occurs.

Time: The time is minimal as far as actually utilizing the homeopathic medicines since they can easily be taken at home in just a minute or two. They also only have to be taken daily or every other day.

The major time commitment will be your visits to a homeopathic practitioner for an initial assessment and periodic check-ups. The first session will probably take from 60 to 90 minutes. Follow-up sessions will probably last between 15 and 45 minutes.

Typically, these visits are scheduled every six to eight weeks at first but may be reduced to only two or three times a year if your child responds well to this treatment. These visits will probably last for one to two years or more.

Convenience: Aside from the recommended visits to a homeopathic practitioner, the actual treatment is very convenient since it usually consists of a single medicine taken once a day or every other day.

Other: Two major advantages that homeopathy has over stimulant medications is that homeopathy has no abuse potential and only a minor side effect of possible short term exacerbation of ADHD symptoms when the homeopathy medicine is first started.

Recommended reading and websites:

Ritalin-Free Kids: Safe and Effective Homeopathic Medicine for ADHD and Other Behavioral and Learning Problems (Revised 2nd edition)
Authors: Judyth Reichenberg-Ullman, N.D., M.S.W. & Robert Ullman, N.D.
Three Rivers Press Copyright 2000
This is an easy-to-read book that explains homeopathy in clear and understandable terms. It includes examples of success stories and provides answers to commonly asked questions about using homeopathy in the treatment of ADHD. It is definitely a valuable book to have as a resource if you are considering using homeopathy.

www.homeopathic.com—Homeopathic Education Services

www.homeopathy.org—National Center for Homeopathy

www.healthy.net/clinic/therapy/homeopat—Health World Online: Homeopathy Center

Contact information:

Homeopathic Educational Services
2124B Kittredge St.
Berkeley, CA 94704
Phone: (510) 649-0294
E-mail: mail@homeopathic.com

National Center for Homeopathy
801 N. Fairfax Street, Suite 306
Alexandria, VA 22314
Phone: (703) 548-7790
E-mail: info@homeopathic.org

12

Essential Nutrients as Supplements

* Iron

* Magnesium

* Zinc

* Essential Fatty Acids

* Glyconutrients

* North American Ginseng

* Ginkgo Biloba

* L-Carnitine

The purpose of this chapter is to show evidence of how deficiencies in some nutrients may be contributing to ADHD and how supplementation of some of these nutrients might help to improve it. Due to the nature of these supplements, this chapter is formatted differently. The research discussed here is at times difficult to understand due to the use of technical and sometimes unfamiliar terms. Please do not get lost in trying to understand every aspect of this information. It is here in an effort to make this chapter thorough and complete but it is not necessary to understand it all in order to benefit.

Also, while there are many vitamins, minerals, and herbs that are touted to help with ADHD, the only ones listed here are those that we have found some research to support their use with this condition. Therefore, we are not stating that any supplements not mentioned here are not effective. What we are saying is that we could not find any published research studies on their use with ADHD.

Overview

Essential nutrients are nutrients which our bodies cannot make on their own. Nutrients do not work alone but synergistically, or in conjunction, with other nutrients. The supplements mentioned here are readily available and can usually be obtained from your local health food store, grocery stores, pharmacies, and even the Internet. However, we recommend that you discuss their use with someone who can help you decide what to use, the proper dosage, and how often to use them. Even though these are all natural products, some may have side effects or even adverse reactions with some medications. Overuse may also cause some health-related issues. Therefore, consulting with your doctor, dietitian, or other health-related practitioner before beginning any supplement program is highly recommended.

While you can always start using essential nutrients in supplementing your child's nutritional intake to see if a supplement makes a difference, the preferred way would be to find out if your child is deficient in any specific nutrient. If there is not a deficiency with a particular essential nutrient, then loading your child down with that supplement will probably not have any effect on his/her ADHD symptoms. Aside from that, taking unnecessary supplements will only increase the risk of negative side effects as well as cost you money that could better be spent elsewhere.

A simple blood test by your doctor can tell you the status of many essential nutrients. Hair sample tests can also be utilized to discover if there are deficits with some nutrients. In addition, listed in this chapter are some signs and symptoms that you may observe in your child which are indicators of a deficiency with certain essential nutrients.

In the beginning, our intention was to discuss all available commercial products as well. However, in looking into them, there appear to be very few research studies on commercial products recommended for ADHD. We also found in more than one instance, the Federal Trade Commission or other regulatory agencies have intervened to stop unsubstantiated claims or deceiving practices.

Again, we are not saying that the lack of research proves that these products do not work. In fact they may very well work. However, we are surprised that more research has not been done and published on these fairly expensive products. Since we were unable to find research studies on these products, we really do not know which products work, why they work, or how well they work.

Commercial products usually utilize a combination of essential nutrients and often include other ingredients as well. These may include some of the essential nutrients described in this chapter for which there is research support. If your child is deficient in a particular nutrient which is included in a commercial product, your child may show improvement using that product. However, one cannot be certain if the improvement is due to the combination of their ingredients or simply because your child is getting a needed nutrient. Therefore, it may be cheaper to just buy that particular supplement or make dietary changes.

If you choose to give your child vitamins, minerals, and other supplements, various guidelines are recommended. Among these are the following:

- Avoid supplements that are artificially colored or flavored and/or contain sugar.

- Avoid thinking that "more is better" since some vitamins and minerals are toxic when taken in large doses.

- Try multi-vitamin, multi-mineral, and herbal supplements separately. If your child starts taking them all at once, you won't be able to determine what is helping or hurting.

- Never think that taking supplements eliminates the need for a balanced, healthy diet.[1]

As a final precaution, here are some key points to keep in mind when using dietary supplements:

- Similar to any conventional medicine, a supplement may cause side effects, trigger allergic reactions, or interact with prescription or non-prescription medication or other supplements your child may already be taking.

- Any side effect or interaction with another supplement or medication may worsen other health conditions.

- Dietary supplements may not be standardized in their manufacturing. As a result, how well they work or any side effects they have may differ among brands or even within different lots of the same brand.

- The form of supplement in a health food or grocery store may not be the same as the one used in research.

- Except for vitamins and minerals, the long-term effects of most dietary supplements are unknown.

The U.S. Food and Drug Administration (FDA) does not regulate dietary supplements in the same way it does medication. Therefore, a dietary supplement can be sold with very limited or no research on how well it works or on its safety. Because of this, it is always recommended that you tell your child's physician if you are using a dietary supplement or if you are thinking about combining any dietary supplement with any medication your child may already be taking.

This first research study we describe compares the effectiveness of Ritalin and a dietary supplement containing several nutrients in treating children with ADHD. In the remainder of the chapter, basic information and studies on iron, magnesium, zinc, essential fatty acids, glyconutrients, North American ginseng, Ginkgo biloba, and carnitine are provided.

Note: A list of recommended readings and websites is located at the end of this chapter.

A Comparison Study of Dietary Supplements and Ritalin® in Treatment of ADHD

Twenty children diagnosed with ADHD and ranging in age from 7 to12 years, were treated with either Ritalin or dietary supplements.[2] The 10 children in the stimulant group were prescribed Ritalin, consisting of 5 to 15 mg dosages two to three times daily, by their family physician. A synergistic combination of dietary supplements was prescribed to the other 10 participants by a certified nurse clinical specialist. The supplement regimen consisted of the following: a multiple vitamin, a multiple mineral, phytonutrients, essential fatty acids and phospholipids (soy lecithin), probiotics, and amino acids.

The following assessments were used: the Conners' Parent Rating Scale revised long form (CPRS-RL) and the Integrated Visual and Auditory/Continuous Performance Test (IVA/CPT) were both administered before the treatment began. The IVA/CPT, a computerized, standardized test that assessed response inhibition and attention problems, was administered again after four weeks of treatment. The following major test quotients can be obtained from the IVA/CPT: the Full Scale Response Control Quotient (FSRCQ) and the Full Scale Attention Quotient (FSAQ). Essentially the FSRCQ measures impulsivity while the FSAQ measures inattentiveness.

Children in both the Ritalin and supplement groups showed significant improvement in impulsivity as indicated by their post-test scores on the FSRCQ. Increases in attentiveness, as measured by the FSAQ scores, were also found to be significant for both groups. There were no significant differences in the levels of improvement between the two treatment groups. Both treatments were found to be equally effective after four weeks of use.

Iron

Background information:

Iron plays a vital role to our health. Primarily linked with protein to form the oxygen-carrying molecule hemoglobin, iron is found in every human cell. Our bodies contain approximately four grams of iron.

Red blood cells pick up oxygen from the lungs and distribute the oxygen to the various tissues throughout our bodies. The ability of red blood cells to carry oxygen is credited to the presence of iron in the hemoglobin molecule.

If our bodies lack iron, they will produce less hemoglobin, resulting in less oxygen being supplied to our tissues and brain. Iron is also a key element of another protein called myoglobin. Myoglobin, like hemoglobin, is an oxygen-carrying molecule that distributes oxygen to muscle cells, particularly to skeletal muscles as well as to the heart.

Various symptoms may indicate a need for more iron in our bodies. Some of these symptoms or signs include the following: decreased ability to concen-

trate, depression, apathy, headaches, increased susceptibility to infections, diz-
ziness, fatigue, hair loss, and brittle nails.

Several nutrients, such as ascorbic acid (vitamin C), copper, cobalt, and
manganese, increase iron absorption. While amino acids may also improve
iron absorption, high dietary intake of calcium may decrease the absorption of
dietary iron. Caffeine and high-fiber foods may also reduce iron absorption.

Iron is present in the human body in two chemical forms. The iron atom
bonds to two electrons in the ferrous form and the iron atom bonds to three
electrons in the ferric form. Iron is capable of going back and forth between
these two forms. It is this property of iron that allows it to play a role in carrying oxygen as part of hemoglobin. However, this same property makes iron an
active component in oxidation-reduction reactions. This simply means that
iron has the ability to act like a free radical in our bodies and therefore it can
cause significant damage to tissues. Whenever iron is not bound to hemoglobin or to some other carrier protein, it can move throughout the body as free
iron causing damage anywhere it travels.

Since excess iron is not easily eliminated by the body, iron supplementation
should be approached with caution. Most of the iron in our bodies gets recy-
cled. As a result, not only is excess iron toxic, it stays around for a long time
once an individual has a surplus. It appears very likely that excess iron can
aggravate, if not cause, some neurological problems. Therefore, anyone who is
not iron deficient should not take iron supplements when potential risks
might exist and no benefit can be found.

The serum ferritin test, which measures how much iron is stored in the
body, is the best way to determine whether your child is deficient or not. The
results will be low if your child is deficient and high if he or she has an excess
of iron.

If children are deficient in iron, however, there is value in giving them iron
supplements. There are two forms of dietary iron: heme and nonheme. Heme
iron is derived from hemoglobin and is found in red meats, fish, and poultry.
Although heme iron is absorbed better, most dietary supplements contain ferrous sulfate, a source of non-heme iron. Non-heme iron is found in plant food
and dairy products.

There are various forms of supplemental iron. Most supplements have a
10% absorption rate, which means that the body only absorbs 1mg for every
10 mg taken. Ferrochel® has a 75% absorption rate. This iron supplement is
not affected by foods that bind iron. Additionally, since it is amino acid
bound, Ferrochel does not become free iron in the body. Therefore, it does

not have the dangers and side effects of other iron supplements. Ferrochel is the only iron supplement that has been given the "GRAS" (generally regarded as safe) designation by the Federal Drug Administration.

Sources:

- Kane, A. *ADHD and Iron Deficiency*. Retrieved June 3, 2005, from http://www.mental-health-matters.com/articles/print.php?artID=751

- The World's Healthiest Foods. *Iron*. Retrieved July 5, 2005, from http://www.whfoods.com/genpage.php?tname=nutrient&dbid=70

- National Institutes of Health: Office of Dietary Supplements. *Dietary Supplement Fact Sheet: Iron*. Retrieved July 11, 2005, from http://ods.od.nih.gov/factsheets/iron.asp

Research:
Iron Treatment in ADHD Children

Researchers in Israel examined non-anemic ADHD children in regard to the effect of short-term iron administration on behavior.[1] Participants were 14 boys, ranging in age from 7 to 11, who had all been previously diagnosed with ADHD.

Each participant was given an iron preparation (Ferrocal) for 30 days at a daily dosage of 5 mg/kg. Blood samples, measuring hemoglobin, hematocrit, mean corpuscular hemoglobin concentration, serum iron level, iron-binding capacity, and ferritin levels among other factors, were also taken before and after the treatment period. The blood sample taken after the 30-day treatment period showed a significant increase in serum ferritin levels.

The abbreviated Conners' Rating Scale was completed by parents and teachers prior to the start of the treatment and 30 days after the treatment to measure the severity of the children's ADHD symptoms. While a significant decrease in the parents' scores on the Conners' scale was reported after the treatment, indicating an improvement in ADHD symptoms, the teachers' scores on the rating scale remained essentially unchanged.

Iron Deficiency in ADHD Children

The purpose of this study, conducted by a team of medical doctors in France, was to investigate whether iron deficiency contributes to ADHD symptoms in children, as compared to children without ADHD who were matched on age and gender.[2] There were 53 children (45 boys and 8 girls), ranging in age from 4 to 14 years, in the ADHD group. The control group consisted of 27 children (20 boys and 7 girls) without ADHD who ranged in age from 5 to 15 years.

The Conners' Parent Rating Scale (CPRS), with its hyperactivity, cognitive, and oppositional subscales, was used to assess the severity of ADHD symptoms. After completing the CPRS, serum ferritin levels were measured in all participants. Blood hemoglobin, hematocrit, and iron levels were also evaluated.

Results showed that the average serum ferritin levels were lower in the ADHD children than in the control group; in fact, the serum ferritin levels in the ADHD children were twice as low as in the children without ADHD whose levels were within the normal range. For one third of the ADHD children, their serum ferritin levels were considered to be in the extremely low range. The serum iron, hemoglobin, and hematocrit levels, however, were within normal ranges in both groups of children.

According to the researchers, since hemoglobin and hematocrit levels were normal for the ADHD group, it was possible to rule out anemia. Therefore, the findings indicated that low ferritin levels need to be considered as a specific abnormality, even though the reason for the low level in the ADHD children was unclear.

Low serum ferritin levels were associated with more severe general ADHD symptoms as measured by the CPRS. One of the key findings was that serum ferritin levels were inversely correlated with the severity of ADHD. Children who were most severely iron deficient were the most inattentive, impulsive, and hyperactive.

Of the three subscales of the CPRS, only the cognitive subscale score correlated significantly with low ferritin levels. This finding suggests the children who are iron deficient are primarily inattentive and distractible and suffer from learning disabilities. Additionally, there was also a trend toward a correlation between the hyperactivity subscale score and serum ferritin levels, with those who were more severely deficient displaying increased motor restlessness.

In the final section of the article, the researchers briefly connected their results to other research studies. They reiterated that a causal relationship between iron deficiency and poor cognitive development and/or behavorial problems has been well documented over the past 30 years. Low ferritin levels in children have been reported to affect the development of the central nervous system, leading to such conditions as behavioral disorders.

In the brain, iron is bound to ferritin, the levels of which are increased by iron supplementation and decreased by iron deficiency. According to the researchers, the results of this study suggest that low iron stores contribute to ADHD and that children with ADHD may benefit from iron supplementation, if they are iron deficient.

Magnesium

Background information:

Magnesium is often referred to as a "macromineral," since our diets must provide us with hundreds of milligrams of magnesium daily. Magnesium is primarily found in the bones (60-65%) and the muscles (25%) of our bodies. Like all minerals, magnesium cannot be made by the body. Consequently, we must get a sufficient supply of magnesium from our diet and/or supplements in order to remain healthy.

This "macromineral" is vital for growth and development, immune system function, nervous and cardiovascular health, and the absorption of calcium. It is also necessary for nerve impulse conduction and muscle contraction. Without magnesium, the production of cellular energy ceases and the electrical stability of our cells wanes.

Magnesium is essential for strong bones, cardiac function and conductivity, neurochemical transmission, and skeletal muscle relaxation. It is also vitally important for maintaining normal intracellular calcium, potassium, and sodium levels. In addition, this mineral has also been identified as essential in over 300 enzyme reactions within the human body.

The metabolic role of magnesium is so diverse that it is extremely difficult to find any body system which is not affected by a lack of magnesium. In fact, our cardiovascular system, digestive system, nervous system, endocrine system, muscles, kidneys, liver, and brain are all directly dependent on magnesium for healthy metabolic functioning.

Various symptoms may indicate a lack of magnesium. Some of these signs or symptoms are: headaches; softening and/or weakening of bones; muscle weakness, tremors, or spasms; depression; seizures; nausea or vomiting; lack of appetite; heart arrhythmia or elevated heart rate; elevated blood pressure; and imbalanced blood sugar levels.

On the other hand, taking too much magnesium may lead to abdominal cramping and diarrhea. Even more serious side effects can develop with excessive doses through taking laxatives and antacids which contain magnesium. Signs of excessive magnesium are similar to signs of deficiency and may include nausea, diarrhea, appetite loss, muscle weakness, difficulty breathing, and irregular heartbeat. Generally, the amounts of magnesium found in nutritional supplements, however, are not likely to cause such problems.

Magnesium is available as a dietary supplement in one of two forms—chelated or non-chelated. The term "chelated" means connected with another molecule. For magnesium, amino acid chelates are the most common chelates. In this case, magnesium is attached to a building block of protein, called an amino acid. Magnesium glycinate, magnesium aspartate, and magnesium taurate are the most widely available. The non-chelated forms of magnesium include magnesium sulfate, magnesium oxide, and magnesium carbonate. Some research evidence indicates that chelated forms may be better absorbed by the body than non-chelated forms.

Sources:

- The World's Healthiest Foods. *Magnesium*. Retrieved July 5, 2005, from http://whfoods.com/genpage.php?tname=nurtrient&dbid=75

- National Institutes of Health: Office of Dietary Supplements. *Dietary Supplement Fact Sheet: Magnesium*. Retrieved July 11, 2005, from http://ods.od.nih.gov/factsheets/magnesium.asp

- Lininger Jr., S.W., Gaby, A., Austin, S., Brown, D., Wright, J., & Duncan, A. (1999). *The natural pharmacy: Complete home reference to natural medicine* (2nd ed.). New York: Three Rivers Press.

Research:
Assessing Magnesium Levels in ADHD Children

Researchers in Poland investigated the magnesium levels in the blood serum, red blood cells, and hair of 116 children diagnosed with ADHD.[1] Participants (96 boys and 20 girls) ranged in age from 9 to 12 years. The levels of magnesium in the ADHD children were compared with magnesium concentration in serum and in hair samples of identified healthy children without ADHD. While approximately 20% to 50% of healthy children in two separate studies exhibited magnesium deficiency, 95% of the ADHD children were found to have a magnesium deficiency. In this study, magnesium deficiency occurred in hair in 78% of the ADHD children, in red blood cells in 59%, and in blood serum in 34%.

The researchers concluded that magnesium deficiency is found more often in ADHD children than in children without ADHD. The researchers also examined whether co-existing conditions, such as conduct disorder, opposi-tional defiant disorder, tics, separation anxiety, or bedwetting, had any impact on the percentage of magnesium deficiency in the ADHD children. Results showed that magnesium deficiency occurs in children with ADHD indepen-dently of other co-existing conditions.

Effect of Magnesium Supplementation on Hyperactivity

This research was conducted by the same team of Polish scientists as the pre-viously described investigation. In the study 50 ADHD children (ages 7 to 12) recognized as having a magnesium deficiency, were assigned to a six-month trial of magnesium supplementation (200 mg per day) in addition to their usual treatment regimen.[2] Another group of 25 ADHD children were assigned to the same treatment regimen without magnesium.

Assessment instruments used to measure changes in hyperactivity were the Conners' Rating Scale for Parents and Teachers, Wender's Scale of Behavior, and the Quotient of Development to Freedom from Distractibility.

At the end of the six months, the children taking the magnesium supple-ment showed a significant reduction in their ADHD symptoms as compared to the group whose treatment did not include magnesium therapy. Parents and teachers ratings on the Conners' scale and ratings on the Wender's Scale indicated that the behavior of the children in the magnesium supplement group had shown improvement after receiving the supplements. In contrast, scores for the children in the group not receiving the magnesium treatment did not improve on either of these assessments; in fact an intensification of clinical symptoms of hyperactivity occurred. Finally, while the group receiving no magnesium did not improve on the distractibility measure, the children receiving the magnesium supplement showed improved scores on the freedom from distractibility assessment.

Not surprisingly, at the end of the six-month period, the hair samples of the supplement group showed an increase in magnesium contents, as com-pared to the group not receiving the supplement. According to the researchers, the results of their work support the use of magnesium supplementation in combination with traditional treatment for ADHD children.

This study was also reviewed by David Rabiner in the June 1999 issue of *Attention Research Update*. Dr. Rabiner stated that the findings of this study suggest that using a magnesium supplement may be a worthwhile approach in ADHD children who have been identified as deficient in magnesium.[3] At this time, however, the percentage of the ADHD population with such a deficiency is not known. He cautioned against providing extra magnesium to children who were not deficient in magnesium, since there is some evidence from animal studies that doing so could have an adverse effect.

Dr. Rabiner's review also pointed out that this study was not a placebo-controlled double-blind trial, but rather should be considered an "open" trial. The parents and teachers in the study were aware of which children were receiving the magnesium supplements and which were not. Knowing such information has the potential to affect the ratings or outcome that both the teachers and parents reported.

Zinc

Background information:

Zinc is an essential mineral which is only needed in very small amounts in our diets. Although only 50 milligrams or less of zinc is needed by the body on a daily basis, this "micromineral" is very important to many bodily functions. For example, zinc is instrumental in regulating genetic activities, supporting blood sugar balance and metabolic rate, supporting smell and taste sensitivity, and supporting the healthy functioning of our immune system.

There are several symptoms which may indicate zinc deficiency. Some signs of a lack of zinc include: impaired sense of taste and smell, depression, growth failure in children, lack of appetite, and frequent colds and infections.

Taking excessive amounts of zinc may impair the body's immune system and reduce the body's levels of HDL, or good cholesterol. Some additional side effects may be severe nausea and vomiting. In 2001, the National Academy of Sciences established the upper levels (UL), or highest intake, for zinc associated with no adverse health effects for infants, children, and adults.

Since our bodies cannot absorb zinc unless it is first linked with other substances, many manufacturers have produced dietary supplements containing zinc that are referred to as being in a "chelated" (connected with another molecule) form. For zinc, the most common chelates fall into two categories: organic acids and amino acids. Supplemental zinc is also available in an inorganic or non-chelated form. Zinc sulfate and zinc oxide are two examples of the non-chelated form.

Sources:

- The World's Healthiest Foods: Essential Nutrients. *Zinc.* Retrieved July 5, 2005, from http://www.whfoods.com/genpage. php?tname=nutrient&dbid=115

- National Institutes of Health: Office of Dietary Supplements. *Dietary Supplement Fact Sheet: Zinc.* Retrieved July 11, 2005, from http://ods.od.nih.gov/factsheets/zinc.asp

- Lininger Jr., S.W., Gaby, A., Austin, S., Brown, D., Wright, J., & Duncan, A. (1999). *The natural pharmacy: Complete home reference to natural medicine* (2nd ed.). New York: Three Rivers Press.

Research:
Turkish Study Investigates ADHD Link to Free Fatty Acids and Zinc

This study evaluated the relationships between serum free fatty acids (FFA) and zinc and ADHD. The FFA and zinc levels of 48 ADHD children (33 boys and 15 girls) were compared with the levels found in 45 healthy children (30 boys and 15 girls) without ADHD.[1]

Results showed that the serum FFA and zinc levels in the ADHD group were significantly lower than those found in the children without ADHD. The average zinc level in the ADHD group was approximately 43% lower than in the non-ADHD group while the average fatty acid levels in the ADHD group were 69% lower than in the control group.

A statistically significant correlation between decreased zinc and fatty acid levels was found in the ADHD group, but not in the group of children without ADHD. According to the researchers, this finding suggested that fatty acid deficiencies may be secondary to zinc deficiencies in causing ADHD. The researchers therefore concluded that deficiencies in zinc and fatty acids may play a role in the development of ADHD.

Zinc Used in Combination with Methylphenidate to Treat ADHD

This study, conducted in Iran, assessed the effectiveness of zinc sulfate used in conjunction with methylphenidate in the treatment of ADHD.[2] Participants were 44 Iranian children (26 boys and 18 girls) ranging in age from 5 to 11 who had been previously diagnosed with the combined subtype of ADHD. None of the participants had received any stimulant medication prior to enrolling in this study. The children were randomly assigned to either (1) the methylphenidate plus zinc treatment group or (2) the methylphenidate plus placebo group for a six-week double blind clinical trial. The dosage of zinc sulfate was 55 mg per day; the placebo group received 55 mg of sucrose.

A number of side effects were studied throughout the clinical trial. Similar numbers of children in both treatment groups reported the following side effects: anxiety, decreased appetite, difficulty falling asleep, and headaches. Nausea and abdominal pain were observed more often in the zinc group. Only children in the zinc group (over 50%) reported experiencing a metallic taste in their mouths.

The assessment measure used to determine the effectiveness of the treatment was the Teacher and Parent ADHD Rating Scale, which has been used extensively in Iran in school-age children to provide a valid measure of behavioral abnormality and attention. Both treatment groups showed a significant improvement at the end of the treatment period, as reported by both parents and teachers, when compared to their pre-treatment scores.

The improvement scores for the stimulant medication plus zinc group, however, were significantly greater than those for the medication plus placebo group. This finding led the researchers to conclude that zinc may be beneficial as a supplementary medication in the treatment of ADHD children. The researchers further suggested that ADHD children with a zinc deficiency might benefit from a change in diet or from a therapeutic trial with a zinc supplement.

Zinc Sulphate Reduced ADHD Symptoms in Turkish Children

A team of researchers in Turkey randomly assigned 400 children (72 girls, 328 boys) to either a zinc or a placebo treatment group to study the effectiveness of zinc for ADHD symptoms.[3] The double blind treatment was conducted for a 12-week time period. The average age of the participants was nine years old. Data from all 400 children were used in evaluating the safety of zinc, and data from 95 and 98 participants in the respective treatment groups were used in evaluating the effectiveness.

The daily dose of zinc sulfate was 150 mg and it contained approximately 40 mg of zinc. This dosage remained constant for the 12 weeks of the study. Both the zinc sulfate and the placebo were orally administered by being mixed with fruit juice or other breakfast drink. Which children were receiving zinc sulfate or the placebo was not known by the parents, the teachers, or the children themselves.

Assessment instruments used in the study were the Attention Deficit Hyperactivity Disorder Scale (ADHDS), the Turkish Adaptation of the Conners' Teacher Questionnaire (TACTQ), and the DuPaul Parent Ratings of ADHD. The ADHDS, developed by the researchers, consisted of 46 questions that focused on the following four subscales: attention deficiency, hyperactivity, impulsivity, and impaired socialization. It was administered prior to the beginning of the study, after week 1, after week 4, and after week 12. Both the TACTQ (with its attention deficit, hyperactivity, and conduct subscales) and the DuPaul were given prior to the beginning of the study and at the end.

Additionally, measures of zinc in the bloodstream of the participants were collected prior to the study and after week 1, after week 4, and after week 12. This was done to determine whether initial zinc levels predicted treatment response, and whether zinc levels increased with the treatment, as expected.

Children treated with zinc sulfate demonstrated significant improvement in the total ADHDS score, as compared to the placebo-treated participants by week 4. This improvement was maintained throughout the entire 12-week trial period. By week 12, the participants in the zinc group showed significant improvement in three of the four subscales of the ADHDS as compared to the placebo treated group. These improvements were on the hyperactivity, impulsivity, and impaired socialization subscales. Additionally, significant improvement was shown by the zinc group on the hyperactivity and conduct subscales of the teacher questionnaire. In regard to the changes in scores on the attention deficit subscale of the teacher questionnaire and the DuPaul Parent Rating scale, although there were differences between the treatment groups, the differences were not significant.

Factors predicting a favorable response to the zinc treatment were examined. According to the researchers, the zinc therapy was most effective for the older children with high body mass index (BMI) scores who showed low zinc and low free fatty acid (FFA) levels prior to treatment. During the study, as expected, blood levels of zinc increased for the zinc group but not for those receiving the placebo.

Overall, the zinc sulfate treatment was well tolerated and had a low rate of side effects. The most common side effect reported was a metallic taste in their mouths. A very small number (eight or less) of participants in both treatment groups reported some nausea, vomiting, and abdominal pain.

This particular study was reviewed in the March 2004 issue of *Attention Research Update*. It was described as the first placebo-controlled, double-blind study on the effectiveness of zinc supplementation as a treatment for ADHD. In his newsletter, Dr. Rabiner pointed out that prior research has shown that individuals with ADHD have lower zinc levels than individuals without ADHD. Furthermore, zinc deficiency is also a contributing factor to hyperactivity and impaired concentration. Although the percentage of children with ADHD who have a zinc deficiency is unknown, it appears as though zinc supplementation could be beneficial for some children diagnosed with ADHD.[4]

Essential Fatty Acids

Background information:

Fatty acids are the building blocks of fat in our diet. There are three types of fatty acids: saturated, polyunsaturated and monounsaturated. Omega-3 and omega-6 fatty acids are polyunsaturated fatty acids, which we call "essential" fatty acids. The brain is composed of 60% fats, and most of this fatty tissue is found in the membranes that envelop neurons. Just as the human body is 75% water and therefore requires a daily supply of water to survive, the brain requires essential fatty acids to order to function optimally.

Essential fatty acids (EFAs) are particularly important molecules of what we consider "good" fats which must be consumed in our diets since our bodies are unable to manufacture them. It is also important to know that your body cannot make omega-3 fatty acids from omega-6 fatty acids or omega-6 fatty acids from omega-3 fatty acids.

EFAs help form the membranes of all cells in our body. The body uses omega-3 and omega-6 fatty acids to manufacture prostaglandins. Prostaglandins (PGs) help cells communicate with one another.

Omega-3 essential fatty acids, eicosapentanoic acid (EPA) and docosohex-anoic acid (DHA), are especially important in normal brain function. EPA and DHA are found naturally in fish oil. Major food sources of omega-3 fatty acids include fish and fish oils, dark green leafy vegetables, and some seeds and nuts. Flaxseed oil is also an excellent source of omega-3s.

Omega-6 fatty acids (AA) and DHA are more concentrated in the brain and retina than in other cells of the body. In addition to playing a critical role in brain and nerve functioning, they are vital for proper functioning of the immune system. Omega-6 fatty acids are mainly found in vegetables, cereal products, fat spreads, and meats.

Various physical signs are associated with deficiencies in these essential fatty acids. These symptoms include the following:

- excessive thirst

- frequent urination

- rough, dry, or flaky skin

- dry, dull, or unmanageable hair

- dandruff

- soft or brittle, splitting nails

- raised bumps on the skin, particularly on the backs of the arms, elbows, or thighs (known as follicular hyperkeratosis).

If your child displays two or more of these symptoms, your child's health and behavior may benefit by increasing foods rich in EFAs in his/her daily diet and/or by taking EFA supplements. EFAs are essential for your child's optimal health. Being deficient in these essential fatty acids has been found to be a factor in some children with ADHD.

Some individuals may experience increases in blood sugar and cholesterol levels when taking fish oil. There appears to be a connection between the amount of fish oil taken and the increased blood sugar levels. Taking several grams of fish oil causes some people to have more gastrointestinal upsets and to burp up a "fishy" smell. In addition, since EPA and DHA reduce blood clotting, taking them may lead to nose bleeds in some cases.

Most of the safety information regarding Gamma-Linolenic Acid (GLA) comes from studies done with evening primrose oil. Several thousands of individuals have taken evening primrose oil or GLA in scientific studies with no significant adverse side effects reported. The maximum dosage of GLA for young children, however, has not yet been established. Omega-6 supplements, including GLA, should not be used if an individual suffers from a seizure disorder since these supplements appear to induce seizures.

There appear to be very few if any drug or nutrient interactions with flaxseeds or flaxseed oil, which are rich in essential fatty acids. However, individuals with a bowel obstruction of any kind should not take flaxseeds or flaxseed oil.

Sources:

- Zimmerman, M. (1999). *The A.D.D. nutrition solution.* New York: Henry Holt and Company.

- Stevens, L. (2005, July). *The ADD/ADHD Online Newsletter*, 5-6. Retrieved July 4, 2005, from http://users.nlci.com/nutrition/news.htm

- Stevens, L. (2000). "Add essential fatty acids to your child's diet", pp. 83-91, in *12 effective ways to help your ADD/ADHD child.* New York: Avery.

- Lininger Jr., S.W., Gaby, A., Austin, S., Brown, D., Wright, J., & Duncan. A. (1999). *The natural pharmacy: Complete home reference to natural medicine* (2nd ed.). New York: Three Rivers Press.

- University of Maryland Medical Center. *Gamma-Linolenic Acid (GLA).* Retrieved July 11, 2005, from http://www.umn.edu/altmed/ConsSupplement/GammaLinolenicAcidGLAcs.html

- WholeHealthMD Supplements. *Flaxseed Oil.* Retrieved July 11, 2005, from http://www.wholehealthmd.com/refshelf/substances_view/1,1525,783,00.html

Research:
Essential Fatty Acid Levels in Boys with Behavior, Learning, and Health Problems

This study compared the behavior, learning, and health problems of boys with low total omega-3 or total omega-6 fatty acid levels with boys having higher levels of these two essential fatty acids.[1] Ranging in age from 6 to 12 years, the

100 volunteers may or may not have demonstrated symptoms of ADHD or have been formally diagnosed with ADHD.

Data were gathered through the Conners' Parent and Teacher Rating Scales, a health questionnaire, and a blood test. Boys having lower levels of omega-3 fatty acids displayed a significantly greater frequency of three out of seven symptoms associated with EFA deficiencies, as reported by their parents on the health questionnaire. These symptoms were increased thirst, frequent urination, and dry skin. The total EFA deficiency score was also significantly greater for those participants with lower total omega-3 fatty acid levels. Although not every child with ADHD had lower levels of critical EFAs in their blood, about 40% had both lower levels of essential fatty acids and increased symptoms of EFA deficiency.

On the Conners' Parent Rating Scale, participants with lower omega-3 fatty acids scored higher on the following areas: anxiety, conduct, hyperactivity/impulsivity, and the hyperactivity index. Those with lower essential fatty acid levels also displayed more frequent and excessive temper tantrums, problems getting to sleep, and problems waking up in the morning. This same group also had more complaints of frequent stomach aches.

According to the Conners' Parent Rating Scale, the boys with lower omega-3 fatty acid levels also displayed significantly more learning problems than those with higher omega-3 levels. Although no significant differences were found on any of the Conners' Teacher Rating Scale scores dealing with behavior between the lower and higher omega-3 groups, the teachers' evaluation of academic skills in math and overall academic ability were significantly lower for the boys with lower omega-3 fatty acid levels. No significant differences were reported in reading or handwriting.

No significant differences in behavior and learning were found for participants based upon their total omega-6 fatty acid levels. However, differences in several health-related problems were documented for this group. Those with lower total omega-6 levels displayed greater frequencies of dry skin and dry hair, reported having more colds, and recorded using antibiotics more often.

Effects of Efamol® Supplementation in Hyperactive Children

This double-blind, placebo-controlled study, conducted in New Zealand, involved using omega-6 fatty acids in the form of evening primrose oil (Efamol®).[2] The 31 participants (27 boys and 4 girls) were randomly assigned to either the Efamol or the placebo group.

Each child was given three capsules, twice daily. Each EFA capsule contained 360 mg of linoleic acid and 45 mg of gamma-linoleic acid; the placebo capsules contained 500 mg of liquid paraffin. In this cross-over design, half of the children received the placebo for the first four weeks, followed by four weeks of the evening primrose oil. Conversing, the other participants received the omega-6 supplementation first, followed by four weeks of the placebo.

A variety of cognitive, motor, and standardized rating scale measures were used with participants being assessed at the following intervals: (1) prior to treatment, (2) after the second week within the treatment, and (3) after the fourth week of the treatment. Blood samples were also taken prior to the beginning of the treatment and at the end of each four-week treatment phase to determine whether supplementation resulted in any measurable changes to EFA levels.

For the supplement group, significant improvements were shown on only two parent-rated symptoms, attention and motor excess. No significant improvements were shown on any teacher-rated items. Accuracy of short-term memory was the only performance task displaying a significant improvement for the treatment group. Therefore, it was concluded that the evening primrose supplement produced minimal improvements in hyperactive children who were selected without regard to their baseline EFA levels.

Discussion

In a 2004 article reviewing clinical trials of fatty acid treatment in ADHD, two critical shortcomings associated with this study and another early study which also used evening primrose oil were described. The first issue identified was that participants were not chosen for their low fatty acid levels. The second concern was the short length of the treatment period. According to the author, more recent studies have shown that dietary supplementation for a minimum of three months is necessary in order to restore essential fatty acids to normal levels. The full crossover design, which both studies employed, was also problematic. Having participants switch (crossover) from treatment to placebo or vice versa in the short timeframe of four weeks did not allow sufficient time for the effect of the supplementation to be measured.[3]

Effects of Highly Unsaturated Fatty Acids on ADHD-Related Symptoms

This study, conducted in Ireland, investigated the effects of highly unsaturated fatty acids (HUFAs) on ADHD-related symptoms in children with a specific learning disability in reading.[4] Although none of the 41 participants, 35 boys and 6 girls, were formally diagnosed with ADHD, all of them scored above-average for high levels of ADHD symptoms based on parent responses to the Conners' Parent Rating Scale (CPRS-L). The children, who ranged in age from 8 to 12 years, were randomly assigned to either receive HUFA supplementation (containing both omega 3 and omega 6 fatty acids) or an identical-looking placebo (containing olive oil) for a 12-week treatment period. Dosages were eight capsules daily for 12 weeks for both the supplement and placebo groups. Neither the parents nor the children themselves were aware of which treatment they were receiving.

The Conners' Parent Rating Scale, administered prior to the start of the study and at completion, was used to assess the effectiveness of the supplementation treatment. The Conners' evaluation instrument has the following seven subscales which assess individual features of ADHD: oppositional, cognitive problems, hyperactivity, anxious/shy, perfectionism, social problems, and psychosomatic. It also has these seven global scales: ADHD index, restless-impulsive, emotional lability, global index, DSM inattention, DSM hyperactive/impulsive, and DSM global total. The HUFA and placebo groups did not differ on any of the Conners' subscales prior to the supplement treatment.

In comparing the two groups after 12 weeks, the supplement group had significantly lower scores on the DSM inattention and the global total subscales as well as a trend toward lower scores on the restless-impulsive subscale. Within the placebo group, no significant improvements were found on any subscale after the 12-week treatment, and on one global scale, the ADHD index, their scores indicated a significant deterioration. Among the children receiving the omega 3 and omega 6 fatty acids, statistically significant reductions in ADHD symptoms were found in the following areas: psychosomatic problems, cognitive problems, anxiety/shy, attention problems, hyperactivity, and the global index measuring a wide range of behavioral problems.

Discussion

This double-blind, placebo-controlled pilot study was reviewed in the June 2002 issue of *Attention Research Update*. Results were described as impressive; however, several of the study's limitations were also addressed.

One of the limitations cited was that none of the participants had been formally diagnosed with ADHD, although all of them had elevated ADHD symptoms prior to beginning treatment. Therefore, the question of whether similar effects would be found in ADHD-diagnosed children, without a reading disability, was raised. Another point raised was that no blood sampling had been taken, so it was unclear as to whether the participants had fatty acid deficiencies to start with, or whether the supplementations actually raised the fatty acid levels of the children. Interestingly, Dr. Rabiner was clear to point out that since participants were not selected because of their low fatty acid levels, the results of the study were even more noteworthy. Finally, although additional studies involving more children clinically diagnosed with ADHD are needed, this study's results indicate that highly unsaturated fatty acids have potential as a helpful intervention for children with ADHD.[5]

Using Fatty Acid Supplementation with Developmental Coordination Disorder

This study, conducted in England, involved 117 children diagnosed with Developmental Coordination Disorder (DCD).[6] Although many of the participants, ranging in age from 5 to 12 years, had elevated levels of ADHD symptoms, they were not formally diagnosed with ADHD; none of the participants were receiving any treatment for their condition prior to beginning the study. Even though DCD is a different disorder from ADHD, children with DCD often experience similar issues in school, such as difficulty with organization skills, attention, and behavioral problems.

Participants (78 boys and 39 girls) were randomly assigned to either the dietary fatty acid supplementation treatment group or the placebo group. The initial treatment phase lasted for three months. At the end of three months, children in the treatment group continued to receive fatty acid supplementation for an additional three months while those in the placebo group were switched to the fatty acid supplements.

The fatty acid supplements contained 80% fish oil and 20% evening primrose oil in the form of gelatin capsules. The daily dosage consisted of six capsules, with two taken in the early morning, two at lunch, and the remaining two in the late afternoon. The supplement treatment provided omega-3 fatty acids, omega-6 fatty acids, and a natural form of vitamin E. The placebo consisted of olive oil capsules. Teachers administered the capsules during the week while parents were responsible for administering them on the weekend.

Several assessment measures were collected prior to the beginning of the study, at the three-month mark, and after six months to determine whether the fatty acid supplementation was effective. Instruments used were the Conners' Teacher Rating Scale, Long Version (to measure ADHD-related symptoms), the Wechsler Objective Reading Dimensions (to measure reading and spelling achievement), and the Movement Assessment Battery for Children (to measure motor functioning).

After three months, children in the supplement treatment group showed a significant decline in ADHD-related symptoms (hyperactivity, restless/impulsive behaviors, inattention, opposition, cognitive problems, and anxiety), while scores for children in the placebo group were basically unchanged. Within the supplement group, 16 children had initially scored in the "elevated" symptom range prior to beginning treatment; after three months, seven of these participants no longer scored in this higher level range. In contrast, only one of the 16 participants in the placebo group showed this same improvement.

Prior to treatment, children in both groups were about one year behind their peers in both reading and spelling achievement scores. After three months, statistically significant gains were shown by the fatty acid group. Their gains averaged 9.5 months in reading and 6.6 months in spelling while those in the placebo group gained only 3.3 months in reading and 1.2 months in spelling.

At the end of six months (when the original placebo group had been taking the supplement for three months), assessments were administered a final time. Results indicated that ADHD symptoms declined significantly for the placebo group who had taken the supplement for three months; scores for those children who had received the supplement throughout the six-month period also continued to show improvement. Additionally, no adverse side effects were reported.

Reading and spelling gains were shown in both groups at the end of the six months. Scores for those in the supplement group increased an additional 10.9 months in reading and 5.3 months in spelling. Participants in the group who had switched to the supplement at the three-month mark showed an average gain of 13.5 months in reading and 6.2 months in spelling.

Motor functioning gains, however, were only modest at the end of three months and again at six months. There were no significant differences between the two treatment groups.

According to the researchers, further studies are needed to determine the optimal dosage as well as the optimal combination of fatty acids. They believe the specific amounts of omega-3 and omega-6 fatty acids are critical as well as the ratio of EPA to DHA.

Discussion

This double-blind, placebo controlled study is highlighted in the June 2005 issue of *Attention Research Update*. In his review, Dr. Rabiner described the results as exciting and positive. He emphasized that this research project was carefully conducted, with the children, teachers, and parents all unaware as to when the participants were receiving the fatty acid supplementation and when they were receiving the placebo. Due to these strict controls, the benefits reported can be safely attributed to the effects of the fatty acid supplementation. However, since the participants were not diagnosed with ADHD, even though many did show elevated levels of ADHD symptoms, Dr. Rabiner recommended that additional research focusing on the effect of fatty acid supplementation on the academic functioning and behavior of ADHD children should be conducted.[7]

EFA Supplementation in Children with Inattention and Hyperactivity

This study assessed the effect of supplementation with polyunsaturated fatty acids (PUFAs) on fatty acid composition and behavior in children diagnosed with ADHD who also reported thirst and skin problems.[8] Fifty participants were randomly assigned to either the PUFA or placebo group for four months. Eighteen participants in the PUFA group and 15 participants in the placebo group completed the study.

Those in the treatment group received eight capsules of the PUFA supplement (Efalex®) per day while the placebo group received eight capsules containing olive oil. Each PUFA capsule contained 60 mg DHA, 10 mg EPA, 5 mg, AA, 12 mg GLA, and 3 mg vitamin E. The children took four capsules with breakfast and four at dinnertime for the entire treatment period. Blood samples were taken to measure fatty acids levels prior to the study, at two months, and again at four months.

Prior to the study and at the completion of the four-month treatment period, the following two primary assessment measures were completed by both parents and teachers: (1) Conners' Abbreviated Symptom Questionnaires (ASQ) and the (2) Disruptive Behavior Disorders (DBD) Rating Scale, which assesses hyperactivity, attention, conduct, and oppositional defiant behavior. The Conners' Continuous Performance Test (CPT) and the revised version of the Woodcock-Johnson (WJ-R) Tests of Cognitive Ability were also used as assessment measures. The CPT, which is a computerized test that measures inattention and impulsivity, lasts for approximately 14 minutes; children with ADHD have a difficult time maintaining attention for the entire time period. The Woodcock-Johnson battery of tests measures factors such as short-term memory, processing speed, auditory processing, and visual processing.

Although few results were statistically significant, two clear improvements for the supplement group were reported. Parents' scores for conduct on the DBD Rating Scale were significantly improved for the PUFA group, but not for the placebo group, and teachers' assessment measures showed significant improvement on the attention subscale of the DBD for the PUFA group only.

Increased DHA, an omega-3 EFA, in the blood was associated with a lowering in the deficiency scores and also with teachers' assessment of attention. Higher EPA, also an omega-3 EFA, was associated with a decrease in the deficiency scores as well as with parents' responses on the questionnaire assessing behavior. Some symptoms of EFA deficiency also improved; there was approximately 50% improvement for dry skin and almost 43% improvement for dry hair. Frequent urination scores also decreased by 30% and excessive thirst scores improved by 33% for the EFA group.

Glyconutrients

Background information:

Glyconutrients are "sweet nutrients" or dietary nutrients that are composed of specific biologically active sugars, which are nontoxic. According to recent scientific research, there are eight simple dietary sugars, or monosaccharides, that form the basic foundation of life at the cellular level. The eight essential saccharides needed for glycoprotein synthesis are: glucose, galactose, mannose, fucose, xylose, N-acetylglucosamine, N-acetylgalactosamine, and N-acetylneuraminic acid. These sugars combine with proteins and fats to create glycoforms which coat the surface of basically every cell in the body. These glycoforms act as cellular recognition molecules by communicating the messages of healthy functioning in the human body. The majority of these eight saccharides, however, are often lacking in the typical modern diet.

Source:

- The Nutrition Science Site: Nutritional Ingredients. Retrieved July 7, 2005, from http://www.glycoscience.org

Research:
*Effect of Glyconutritional Supplements and Phytonutritional Supplements on ADHD**

This six-week study, involving 17 children (3 girls and 14 boys), reported the effects of two nutritional supplements on the severity of ADHD symptoms.[1] The participants, ranging in age from 6 to 14 years, were assigned to one of three treatment groups. Five of the children, who were not taking any medication, were "naturally" assigned to the "No Med" group. The other 12 children, who were already on prescribed doses of methylphenidate, were randomly assigned to either the drug reduction group (Med Red) or the medication (Med) group. While the dosage of the "Med Red" group was cut in half after the first two weeks, the dosage of the participants in the "Med" group remained unchanged throughout the study.

Several assessment instruments, including the DuPaul ADHD rating scale, the Conners' Abbreviated (10-item) Teacher and Parent Rating Scales, and the IOWA-Conners' Scale (a modification of the Conners' scale) were completed by both parents and teachers to determine the effectiveness of the nutritional supplements. In addition, parents completed a Health Benefit Rating Scale, developed by the researchers to identify the "side effects" of the participants. Assessments were completed prior to the beginning of the study as a baseline, after two weeks (when the dosage of the "Med Red" group was cut in half), and again during the fifth and sixth weeks of the study.

Throughout the study, teachers were unaware the children were receiving dietary supplements. However, they were told adjustments might be made in medication dosages and, as a result, it would be necessary for them to complete forms and evaluate the children's behavior at certain intervals.

The treatment began with the children receiving the glyconutritional supplement, containing the eight essential saccharides, for three weeks. The dosage was determined by the weight of each child, with one capsule per every 10 pounds of body weight the first day and one capsule per every 20 pounds of body weight thereafter. The dietary supplements were taken at home as part of meals, mostly after breakfast.

After three weeks, a phytonutritional supplement was added to the treatment regimen. The phytonutritional supplement consisted of the same essential sugars as the glyconutritional supplement, except in lesser amounts. In addition, the added supplement included flash-dried fruits and vegetables, such as carrots, cabbage, broccoli, kale, tomato, papaya, and pineapple. The children received the glyconutritional supplement for the entire six weeks.

The glyconutritional supplement decreased the number and severity of ADHD symptoms, associated Oppositional Defiant Disorder (ODD) symptoms, and Conduct Disorder (CD) symptoms. All groups showed decreases in the ADHD symptoms; these improvements were statistically significant for all parent measures. Interestingly, the greatest decrease in symptoms was noted after two weeks, with little additional change thereafter.

In the discussion section of the article, the researchers pointed out these supplements significantly reduced the number and severity of ADHD symptoms, regardless of whether the children were taking or not taking stimulant medication. The researchers did not advocate the elimination of methylphenidate, but rather recommended further studies of naturally occurring food substances that may reduce ADHD symptoms. Using nutritional supplements, which have no significant negative side effects, would provide an option to parents who are uncomfortable with giving their children medications. The researchers also recommended the use of supplements in conjunction with medications to improve health and reduce the side effects of stimulants.

*Mannatech™ Incorporated, a multi-level marketing company, supplied the supplements used in this study. The glyconutritional supplement was Ambrotose® complex and the phytonutritional supplement was Phyto Bears™. The Phyto Bears product is no longer available. It has now been replaced with Manna Bears™, which has been reformulated with increased glyconutrient content.

If you choose to try glyconutrients with your child, you can buy them directly from Mannatech's website, which directs you to an associate's retail web page (Mannapages). You may want to contact an associate as it is beneficial to have assistance in determining the appropriate product and dosages that your child may need.

If you are interested in glyconutrients, more detailed information can be found at the following:

Science Magazine, Special Issue, *Carbohydrates and Glycobiology,* March 23, 2001. (This entire issue was devoted to these sugars.)

www.glycoscience.org
www.glycoinformation.com

Contact Information:
Mannatech Incorporated
600 S. Royal Lane, Suite 200
Coppell, TX 75019
Phone: (972) 471-7400
Website: www.mannatech.com

North American Ginseng
and
Ginkgo Biloba

Background information :

The Latin name for North American ginseng, or American ginseng, is *Panax quinquefolius.* It was discovered in Canada in the 18th century. Over the last 100 years, American ginseng has gained popularity for its therapeutic qualities. Although it is often prepared as a tea, it is also common in single-herb and combination-therapy supplements.

Ginseng contains ginsenosides, which stimulate the body's immune system and fight stress and fatigue. This herb has also been shown to affect the neurotransmitter processes in the brain. It is believed that the primary active components of American ginseng (ginsenosides) may also play a "protector" role in the dopamine system in the brain, providing stress-relieving benefits. Some research studies, using both single and combination herb preparations of North American ginseng, suggest that this herb may help improve cognitive function related to memory quality, response time, as well as accuracy and general memory improvement.

When taken in moderation, American ginseng has an excellent safety profile. Individuals taking large amounts over extended periods of time have reported adverse side effects including headaches, sleeplessness, nervousness, blood pressure changes, and/or hypertension.

Source:

- Clarocet Ingredient Reference Library. *American Ginseng*. Retrieved July 10, 2005, from http://www.clarocet. com/referencelibrary/american-ginseng/index.htm

Ginkgo biloba extract, from the leaves of the Ginkgo biloba tree, has been used for thousands of years in traditional Chinese medicine. An extract of ginkgo biloba extract is used to make the supplement. While ginkgo extract is the most commonly used herbal medicine in Europe, only in the last few decades have the medicinal uses for this herb been studied in the West.

While the benefits of ginkgo may not be totally understood, it appears to improve blood flow in the brain, and throughout the body, by thinning the blood. It also reduces inflammation and acts as an antioxidant to fight cell damage.

Ginkgo has been used to treat several health conditions. Some evidence indicates that ginkgo may be helpful in the treatment of circulatory disorders, memory impairment, concentration problems, anxiety, stress, and mood problems caused by decreased blood flow in the brain.

Although the risk appears to be very low, bleeding problems are the main complication that has been linked to the use of ginkgo. Because ginkgo may reduce the blood's ability to clot, it is not recommended for any individual who is already taking a blood-thinning medication.

Sources:

- Yahoo! Health Encyclopedia. *Ginkgo Biloba*. Retrieved July 11, 2005, from http://health.yahoo.com/ency/healthwise/hw136253spec

- Wholehealthmd Supplements. *Ginkgo Biloba*. Retrieved July 11, 2005, from http://www.wholehealthmd.com/refshelf/substances_view/ 1,1525,788,00.html

Research:

Effect of AD-FX® (extract of North American Ginseng and Ginkgo Biloba) on ADHD

This pilot study, conducted in Canada, used a combination herbal product containing American ginseng extract and Ginkgo biloba extract to investigate its ability to improve ADHD symptoms.[1] Participants were 36 children, ranging in age from 3 to 17 years, whose ADHD diagnosis had been previously confirmed by a physician.

Twenty-five participants were on medication prior to beginning the treatment. These children were encouraged not to change medication or dosage until the study was completed. However, those taking medication were only permitted to participate if their ADHD symptoms were poorly controlled despite being on medication.

Parents received labeled bottles containing 60 capsules of the herbal product AD-FX®, manufactured by CV Technologies in Edmonton, Alberta. Each capsule contained 200 mg of American ginseng extract (*Panax quinquefolium*) and 50 mg of Ginkgo biloba extract. The children were to take one capsule twice daily on an empty stomach, at least 30 minutes before mealtime.

The Conners' Parent Rating Scale (CPRS) was used to assess the effectiveness of the herbal treatment. Parents completed the 80-question revised, longer version (RL) of the CPRS before the study began, after two weeks, and again at the end of the four-week treatment period. The CPRS-RL has seven individual symptom categories and seven global categories. The individual categories are as follows: (1) oppositional, (2) cognitive problems, (3) hyperactive-impulsive, (4) anxious-shy, (5) perfectionism, (6) social problems, and (7) psychosomatic. The global symptom categories are: (1) ADHD index, (2) global index: restless-impulsive, (3) global index: emotional lability, (4) global index: total (5) DSM-IV: inattentive, (6) DSM-IV: hyperactive-impulsive, and (7) DSM-IV: total.

Significant improvement was shown on all seven individual symptom categories at the completion of the four-week treatment period. In fact, after two weeks, 18 (50%) children showed significant improvement on the hyperactive-impulsive category, 20 (56%) on cognitive problems, and 22 (64%) on the oppositional attribute.

There was also a significant improvement on all seven global categories of the Conners' rating scale at both two and four weeks. After four weeks on AD-FX, 53% of the children improved in the inattentive category, 74%

improved on the hyperactive-impulsive attribute, and 53% improved on the restless-impulsive category.

This small pilot study appears to be the first research study to use a combination of American ginseng and Ginkgo biloba to treat ADHD symptoms. While the results suggest that AD-FX is safe and well tolerated and may be helpful in effectively managing behavioral and cognitive difficulties experienced by ADHD children, the researchers do point out that relying only on parental assessment and not having a control group were definite limitations of the study. They recommend further clinical trials of longer duration in the future.

L-Carnitine

Background information:

L-carnitine (or acetyl-L-carnitine)is derived from lysine and methionine, two essential amino acids. Its name comes from the Latin "caro or carnis" meaning flesh or meat. Beef, pork, lamb, poultry, fish, and dairy products are the richest sources of L-carnitine; fruits, vegetables, and grains contain relatively little. Produced in the liver and kidneys, carnitine is used primarily for energy production by way of oxidation, which involves the breakdown of fatty acids for energy.

Over the past decade, scientific research has shown that acetyl-L-carnitine is an important factor in promoting healthy cognitive brain function, as well as in promoting memory maintenance and neurotransmitter production. Clinical trials using acetyl-L-carnitine have shown that this nutrient can be beneficial in treating mental fatigue, including attention concentration. The nutrient may also have some beneficial effect in the area of impulsivity control in the treatment of ADHD.

Generally, L-carnitine appears to be well tolerated and no toxic effects related to an overdose with this nutrient have been reported. However, taking L-carnitine as a supplement may cause mild gastrointestinal symptoms, such as nausea, vomiting, abdominal cramps, or diarrhea, in some cases. Supplements that provide more than 3,000 mg daily may cause an unpleasant "fishy" body odor.

Sources:

- Clarocet Ingredient Reference Library. *Acetyl—L-Carnitine—Clinical references and information for anxiety and ADHD*. Retrieved July 6, 2005, from http://www.clarocet. com/referencelibrary/acetyl-L-carnitine

- The Linus Pauling Institute: Micronutrient Information Center. *L-Carnitine: Toxicity*. Retrieved July 9, 2005, from http://lpi. oregonstate.edu/infocenter/othernuts/carnitine

Research:
Effectiveness of Carnitine on ADHD: Double-blind, Placebo-controlled Study

This double-blind, placebo-controlled study, conducted in the Netherlands, examined the effectiveness of carnitine treatment in children with ADHD.[1] Participants were 24 boys ranging in age from 6 to 13 years who met the criteria for the combined subtype of ADHD according to the DSM-IV.

In this double crossover study, participants were randomly assigned to one of two groups. The treatment order for one group consisted of placebo-carnitine-placebo while the treatment for the other group was carnitine-placebo-carnitine. Each treatment period was eight weeks in length, so the entire study lasted for 24 weeks. The carnitine supplement and placebo were taken twice daily after meals.

Blood samples were taken prior to the study and after each eight-week treatment period. Additionally, participants received a physical examination at screening and in week 24.

Effectiveness of the treatment was assessed by parents completing the Child Behavior Checklist (CBCL) and by teachers completing the 39-item Conners' Teacher Rating Scale. The CBCL is composed of 120 questions with the following subscales: attention problems, delinquency, and aggressive behavior. Each boy was assessed at the end of each of the three trial periods.

Results showed that the school behavior of 13 (out of 24) boys receiving carnitine treatment improved significantly as indicated by the teacher ratings of the Conners' scale. Also, the home behavior of 13 boys receiving the treatment improved significantly as determined by the total score on the CBCL.

Baseline data showed that the participants' scores on both the total CBCL and its three subscales differed significantly from those of normal Dutch boys without ADHD. Treatment with carnitine significantly decreased both the aggressive behavior and the attention problems of these ADHD boys.

There were no adverse side effects observed in a majority of the participants. It was noted that 20 of the 24 boys continued using carnitine after the three trial periods at their parents' request.

As a result of this study's findings, it was concluded that carnitine appeared to be effective and well tolerated for the treatment of a group of ADHD boys who showed significantly abnormal behavior compared to normal Dutch boys prior to beginning treatment. More research studies with larger numbers of children were recommended by the researchers.

A Comment on the "More is Better" Philosophy with Vitamin Therapy

Megavitamin therapy can be defined as taking one or more vitamins in amounts 10 or more times greater than the recommended dietary allowances. The purpose of one research study, involving 41 children (35 boys and 6 girls), was to determine whether megavitamin therapy had positive effects on ADHD children.[1] Participants were enrolled in a two-stage trial. The first stage consisted of a three-month clinical trial of niacinamide, ascorbic acid, pyridoxine, and calcium pantothenate. (Niacinamide is one of the water-soluble B-complex vitamins, ascorbic acid is another name for vitamin C, pyridoxine is another name for vitamin B6, and calcium pantothenate is another name for vitamin B5.) The second stage consisted of four six-week, double-blind, repeated crossover periods.

Findings showed there was no significant difference in most behavioral scores comparing vitamin and placebo treatment during stage two. In general, more positive behavioral responses were observable during placebo treatment as compared with vitamin therapy.

According to the researcher, megavitamins have no beneficial effect for children with ADHD. He concluded that megavitamins are not effective in the management of ADHD and should not be used due to their potentially serious side effects when taken in greater than recommended quantities.

Recommended reading and websites:

12 Effective Ways to Help Your ADD/ADHD Child: Drug-Free Alternatives for Attention-Deficit Disorders

Author: Laura J. Stevens
Avery, a member of Penguin Putnam, Inc. Copyright 2000

The A.D.D. Nutrition Solution
Author: Marcia Zimmerman
Henry Holt and Company Copyright 1999

The Natural Pharmacy: Complete Home Reference to Natural Medicine
Authors: Schuyler W. Lininger, Jr., Alan Gaby, Steve Austin, Donald J.
Brown, Jonathan Wright, & Alice Duncan
Three Rivers Press Copyright 1999

The A-Z Guide to Drug-Herb and Vitamin Interactions
Authors: Schuyler W. Lininger, Jr., Alan Gaby, Steve Austin, Forrest
Batz, Eric Yarnell, Don Brown, & George Constantine
Three Rivers Press Copyright 1999

The ADD/ADHD Online Newsletter: http://www.nlci.com/nutrition
(available free)
Recent topics: ADD/ADHD & iron
            Essential fatty acids & ADHD (four-part series)
            Artificial colors and flavorings
www.ftc.gov/bcp/conline/features/kidsupp.htm—Federal Trade Commission Features
www.wholehealthmd.com

13

Dietary Changes and Food Sensitivities

The extent to which dietary factors may contribute to a child's ADHD symptoms appears to be a topic of continuous debate among parents, healthcare professionals, and researchers. While recognizing that diet may be an important factor for some ADHD children, physicians and researchers have typically minimized the importance of dietary factors for most children with ADHD. On the other hand, many parents believe that diet plays an important factor in their child's behavior and frequently initiate dietary changes, often without the support, and sometimes without the knowledge, of their family doctor.

Large numbers of books have been written that are totally devoted to the subject of nutrition as well as to the relationship between ADHD and nutrition. Going into depth on this extremely broad and complex topic by reviewing countless research studies is beyond the scope of this book. We do, however, recognize that dietary changes can influence the behavior of some children with ADHD. Although not extensive, we have chosen to include what we consider to be valuable information and resources that you as a parent need to be aware of as you decide what is best for your child.

There definitely is research evidence to support the role diet, artificial colors and flavors, and/or food allergies and sensitivities play in regard to symptoms of ADHD. In an effort to assist you in learning more in these areas, we are providing information regarding two free newsletters (*The ADD/ADHD*

Online Newsletter and *Attention Research Update*) that we believe you will find very informative.

For example, Laura Stevens, M.S., focuses on the topics of artificial colors and behavior, food sensitivities, and hidden food allergies in the May, June, and July 2005 issues of her *The ADD/ADHD Online Newsletter*. In each issue, she briefly shares significant research studies that provide evidence of the link between each topic and ADHD in a very readable format. She also provides you with information of symptoms your child might exhibit if he or she has a hidden food allergy and what foods most often provoke an allergic reaction.

The *Attention Research Update* newsletter, authored by Dr. David Rabiner who is a research psychologist at Duke University and which has been referenced in several chapters throughout this book, is another excellent source for a wide range of topics on ADHD. Going to its archives (www.helpforadd.com/archives.htm), you can peruse all of its previous issues. Although its main focus is not diet or nutrition, it provides a relatively short, but clearly written description and summary, of important new research in the field of ADHD in each issue. For example, Dr. Rabiner reviewed the meta-analysis on artificial food colors and ADHD, which is highlighted at the end of this chapter, in the April 2005 issue. As new research is reported in the areas of dietary aspects as they relate to ADHD, this newsletter will likely be a valuable resource to learn more about these research findings.

We would also suggest reading a booklet published by the Center for Science in the Public Interest entitled *Diet, ADHD, & Behavior: A Quarter-Century Review*. This 32-page publication, which was published in 1999, can be downloaded free of charge (www.cspinet.org/diet.html). Shortly after its publication, several experts in the field of diet and behavior recommended that parents and professionals first modify children's diets before they resorted to drug therapy. They also called for the Department of Health and Human Services to consider banning synthetic dyes in foods and other products that are widely consumed by children. Such products would include some varieties of candies, cupcakes, sugary breakfast cereals, vitamin pills, and toothpaste.[1]

While we have reviewed various research studies reporting the findings of each treatment option or therapy in all of the other chapters in this book, here we simply encourage you to read the following review of multiple research studies on artificial food colors to "whet your appetite" (pardon the pun!) for reading more information about different dietary factors. The websites of the newsletters we mentioned earlier, which are provided at the end of the chapter, would be a good starting point. Finally, we certainly encourage you to do further research and reading if you believe your child is among those ADHD children where dietary changes could positively impact his/her behavior and overall wellbeing.

Artificial Food Colors

A meta-analysis, published in the December 2004 issue of the *Journal of Developmental and Behavioral Pediatrics*, analyzed the findings of 15 research studies (219 total participants) that reported the results of the relationship between the consumption of artificial food colors and behavioral changes in ADHD children.[2] A meta-analysis does not look at the individual results of each study, but rather looks for a pattern, which provides a more reliable basis for drawing conclusions about the overall pattern of findings in a particular area of research.

All 15 cases were double-blind, crossover trials which means that participants in each study received two different diets, one that included artificial food colors and one that did not. In all studies those parents, and/or teachers, and/or clinicians who assessed the children's behaviors were not aware of which diet the child was receiving at the time.

According to a review of this study published in the April 2005 issue of *Attention Research Update*, the most important finding from analyzing the 15 studies was that the children's behavior showed a statistically significant improvement when artificial food colorings were eliminated from their diet. The size of the improvement was about one third to one half as large as improvement typically seen when children respond favorably to medication treatment. However, the results from this meta-analysis do provide strong evidence that the behavior of ADHD children can be adversely influenced by dietary factors and that eliminating artificial food colorings will, on the average, result in improvements in their behavior.[3]

Another important finding was that children who had previously demonstrated a responsiveness to artificial food colors, or whose parents believed they were responsive to dietary factors, showed an even greater improvement in their behaviors when the food colors were removed. This finding appears to suggest that parents are sensitive to whether their child's behavior is negatively affected by diet. So, as a parent, don't be afraid to trust your instincts. If you believe your child has these sensitivities, if may be well worth your time to make some dietary changes and monitor the results.

There is one cautionary note, however, to consider for these results. The authors pointed out that only ratings from the parents, and not from the teachers, showed improvement when artificial food colorings were eliminated. Therefore, as a parent, you cannot assume that your child is doing better at school even if you observe improvements in behavior at home.

If you plan to implement a diet free from artificial food colorings, it is very important that both you and your child are comfortable with the idea. It is also essential that you carefully monitor whether improvements you see are being observed by your child's teacher.

Recommended readings and websites:

Jacobson, M.F., & Schardt, D. (1999). *Diet, ADHD & Behavior: A Quarter-Century Review.* Washington, D.C.: Center for Science in the Public Interest.-available online at www.cspinet.org./diet.html

www.nlci.com/nutrition/news.htm—*The ADD/ADHD Online Newsletter*
www.helpforadd.com—*Attention Research Update*
www.helpforadd.com/archives.htm—*Attention Research Update* Archives

14

Environmental Factors

Spending time in the outdoors may play an important role in the treatment of ADHD and/or in the severity of some ADHD symptoms. The idea that exposure to nature might improve a person's ability to attend or focus is based on "attention restoration theory." This theory proposes that there are two types of attention, voluntary and involuntary. Voluntary attention, which is also known as directed attention, is used in situations or tasks that require an individual to be able to sustain focus when it is not inherently easy to do so. Individuals become fatigued after prolonged or intense periods of voluntary attention. On the other hand, since involuntary attention does not require effort, it is relatively easy to do.

In attention restoration theory it is believed that natural environments assist in recovering from the fatigue of directed or voluntary attention. It is proposed that natural environments, in part, draw on involuntary attention rather than directed attention. The idea is that remaining focused or attentive in these "green" settings occurs naturally, without any concentrated effort.

A considerable amount of research has been conducted among non-ADHD individuals that show that certain "symptoms" associated with ADHD, such as inattention, are reduced after being exposed to the outdoors and various natural settings. Many individuals experience a sense of rejuvenation or restoration after spending time in nature. In the following two studies, researchers looked at the connection or relationship between activities in nature and their effect or impact on the symptoms of children who were diagnosed with ADHD.

Research:
Connection between ADHD and Green Play Settings

The study examined the relationship between ADHD children's exposure to nature through leisure activities and their ability to attend or focus.[1] Participants in this study were parents of 96 ADHD children, ranging in age from 7 to 12 years. The parents volunteered to complete a survey that dealt with their child's play settings and activities. In the survey's first section, participants were asked to identify one or two after-school or weekend activities after which they felt their child's inattentive symptoms were improved as well as one or two activities after which their child's symptoms worsened.

In the next section of the survey, parents were given a list of 25 different after-school and weekend activities and were asked to rate each activity in terms of its effect on their child's ability to attend. A total of 11 indoor activities, 6 outdoor activities in man-made settings, and 8 activities in green outdoor spaces were evaluated. The rating scale ranged from 1 to 5, with 1 being "much worse" and 5 being "much better." If an activity received a rating of 3, it was considered "neutral" and indicated that the parents believed their child's problems with attending were not noticeably different after participating in it.

Results indicated that "green" activities consistently received higher ratings than either activities occurring indoors or activities in man-made outdoor settings. These differences were statistically significant.

Next, the researchers considered whether "green" activities with more physical activity, such as playing in a tree house, received higher scores than more passive green activities, such as reading a book in the park. They did not find evidence to support this idea, which means that the benefits of being in green space are the same regardless of the activity.

The researchers also wondered whether certain green space activities might be associated with improvement in attention because these activities were more likely to be preferred by the children. Parents' ratings of their child's preferences, however, did not appear to support this belief. Several activities which were reported to be strongly preferred, such as playing video games or watching television, were observed by parents to result in an increase, and not a decrease, in their child's attention problems.

National Study Investigating Green Spaces as Natural Treatment for ADHD

This national study examined the effect of "green spaces" or natural settings on ADHD symptoms across diverse subgroups of U.S. children, all of whom had been formally diagnosed with ADHD.[2] Participants were 452 parents of ADHD children, who ranged in age from 5 to 18. These parents completed a 20 to 30-minute survey which asked them to rate the after effects of 49 common after-school and weekend activities on their children's ADHD symptoms. Parents rated their children in the following four areas: (1) difficulty in completing tasks, (2) difficulty in remaining focused on unappealing tasks, (3) difficulty in listening to and following directions, and (4) difficulty in resisting distractions. For each activity parents indicated whether their child's symptoms were typically "much worse than usual," "worse than usual," "same as usual," "better than usual," or "much better than usual" for approximately an hour or more after taking part in the activity.

Green outdoor activities were compared with both indoor activities and built outdoor activities. "Green outdoor activities" were considered to be those in a primarily natural setting, such as a park, farm, or simply in a green backyard or neighborhood space. "Built outdoor settings" were those considered to be mostly man-made, such as parking lots, downtown areas, or simply any neighborhood space not having much greenery. An activity such as reading, for example, might take place indoors, in an outdoor setting, or in a built outdoor setting.

Parents were unaware of the purpose of the study. Their ratings, therefore, are not likely to have been biased or influenced by what they considered the researchers were hoping to document regarding the influence of natural settings on ADHD symptoms.

Results showed that the green outdoor activities significantly reduced the symptoms of ADHD more than did either built outdoor activities or indoor activities. These findings were consistent across various subgroups of children. Regardless of numerous factors, such as gender, age, household income, geographical area of the country, or type of community (urban or rural) setting, green outdoor activities were beneficial in reducing ADHD symptoms. Additionally, the benefits for green outdoor activities were consistent among ADHD children with or without hyperactivity, and among those with relatively mild, average, and severe symptoms.

Although the researchers stated that their findings were consistent with other studies reporting the restorative or rejuvenating effect that exposure to natural settings can have on the ability of non-ADHD individuals to focus and attend, they were cautious to note that additional research with ADHD children needs to be conducted so the impact of exposure to natural or green settings can be more carefully assessed. Specifically, its effect on other ADHD symptoms, such as impulsivity, needs to be examined as well as its impact on classroom behavior.

Discussion

Exposure to nature certainly appears to have no adverse effects associated with it. Implementation might be as simple as incorporating "daily doses of green" with your child's already existing treatment routine. Choosing a greener route to school, doing homework at a window with a view of nature, or even doing homework outdoors, are some possibilities to try. Although not ideal, watching videos of natural landscapes might be tried in some cases if daily exposure to green spaces proves impractical. Since spending more time outdoors is both easy to implement and inexpensive, it seems quite reasonable for parents to try this "natural treatment" for ADHD to see whether they notice any benefits for their child.

15

Additional Treatments

* Brain Gym® and Educational Kinesiology

* Imagination Gym™

* The Dore Program

* HeartMath® and Freeze-Framer®

* Hemoencephalographic (HEG) Biofeedback

* Color Therapy or Esogetic Colorpuncture Therapy™

* Craniosacral or Cranial Sacral Therapy (CST)

* Bach Flower Essences or Oral Flower Essences

* BrainTrain Cognitive Training

* The Tomatis® Method

* Bio-Acoustical Utilization Device (BAUD)

* Magnetic Therapy

There are several other treatments or therapies that appear to show promise in treating ADHD, but any independently published research studies concerning their validity are either non-existent or very limited. We have chosen to include them here, along with a brief description and pertinent contact information, should you desire to learn more about them and/or explore their use as an option for your child.

Brain Gym® and Educational Kinesiology

Kinesiology is the study of movement while educational kinesiology is the study and application of natural movement to facilitate learning. Although developmental experts have known that movement enhances learning for over 80 years, Dr. Paul Dennison took this knowledge, in collaboration with his wife Gail, and applied specific movements to develop the concept of Educational Kinesiology (Edu-K) and the Brain Gym movements.

To explain how Edu-K works, the Dennisons describe brain function in terms of the following three dimensions: laterality, focus, and centering. Laterality pertains to the ability to coordinate one side or hemisphere of the brain with the other side, especially in the midfield where the two hemispheres must integrate. For example, in one exercise, the individual is to touch his/her left elbow to his/her right knee and the right elbow to the left knee repetitively, thereby moving across the body's midline. The idea is that this simple movement will help the left and right hemispheres of the brain to communicate. The two hemispheres must work together in order for learning to be successful.

The focus dimension describes the relationship between the back and front lobes or areas of the brain. Focus affects comprehension; attention disorders, such as ADHD, are related to the inability to focus. Centering is the ability to coordinate the top and bottom structures of the brain; it allows the individual to balance emotion with rational thought. Stress can disturb centering.

For the brain to function effectively, connections across the neural pathways throughout the brain must work successfully. Learning and functional disabilities occur when information does not flow freely. The idea behind the 26 Brain Gym movements or exercises is that they stimulate this flow of information within the brain, thereby restoring an individual's ability to learn and function at top efficiency. Even though Brain Gym activities were originally designed for kindergarten through college level students in the classroom, Brain Gym exercises can be practiced at home.

Contact information:

Brain Gym International
1575 Spinnaker Drive, Suite 204B
Ventura, CA 93001
Phone: (800) 356-2109 or (805) 658-7942
E-mail: edukfd@earthlink.net
www.braingym.org

Imagination Gym™

Imagination Gym™ exercises the mind, rather than the muscles, to develop an individual's creative and imaginative side. The Enchanted Forest audio CD, which is used in this therapy, is based on Brain Gym's theory involving the integration of the right and left hemispheres of the brain. The program has been designed for children with ADHD, Asperger's, Oppositional Defiant Disorder (ODD), and related conditions. According to its website, the audio CD is interactive and self-paced. The interaction is said to increase a child's sense of well being as well as to correct behavioral problems.

Since the program is not a test, it does not follow any prescribed timetable. There is also no right or wrong way of listening to "The Enchanted Forest." This audio CD program is designed so that it can be used again and again. Since it is guided, the listener can change the story each time he or she listens.

Information on its website reports that regular use of "The Enchanted Forest" CD helps the ADHD child improve in various areas including the following: concentration and focus, attention to detail, listening skills, following directions, relaxing, sitting still, hyperactivity, social skills, reducing stress, and sleeping more soundly.

Since having an ADHD child affects every member of the family, one unique feature of the CD is its ability to be used by all members of the family to assist with daily tensions and stress. According to its website, research has shown that "The Enchanted Forest" CD can help both child and adults with stress, concentration problems, sleeping problems, imagination, and creativity.

Contact information:

The Imagination Gym Company
9 Willow Business Park
Knockmitten Lane
Dublin 12, Ireland
Phone: 00 353 1 4603193/4603194
E-mail: info@imaginationgym.ws
www.imaginationgym.com

The Dore Program

Current research has shown that the cerebellum, located in the bottom rear portion of the head, is responsible for integrating sensory information to allow efficient learning to occur. However, if the neural pathways or connectors that link the cerebrum, or "linking brain," and the cerebellum are not yet fully developed, the cerebellum is unable to process information quickly enough. This inability to process information efficiently is called cerebellar developmental delay (CDD). The idea behind the Dore method is that the cerebellum can be stimulated to create new neural pathways which speed up the processing of information, and therefore help with learning, language, emotion, and motor skills. Since the brain has plasticity, once the cerebellum has been developed, the idea is that it stays that way. It will not regress.

The Dore program involves an extensive initial assessment visit to determine how the individual's cerebellum has developed. After examining the assessment results, a Dore therapist or professional at a Dore Achievement Center prescribes a personal exercise program. The focus is on physical exercise that stimulates the brain. With the Dore approach, certain physical exercises, usually taking 5 to 10 minutes twice a day, are carried out at home. For example, a typical exercise might be as follows: standing on a cushion on one leg and throwing a beanbag from one hand to another for one minute.

Wynford Dore, from whom the program and centers take their name, established the first treatment center in the United Kingdom in 2000. His original treatment was called Dyslexia Dyspraxia Attention Deficit Treatment. Presently 15 Dore Achievement Centers can be found in the United Kingdom, Australia, and the United States, with more expansion being planned.

Contact information:

Phone: (866) 784-4377
E-mail: info@dorecenters.com
www.dorecenters.com

HeartMath® and Freeze-Framer®

The Freeze-Framer® was developed based on research findings conducted by the Institute of HeartMath® (IHM) in Boulder Creek, California. The IHM's research shows that an individual's state of heart, or "heart entrainment," is integrally linked with his or her state of mind, emotions, and physiology. The Freeze-Framer Interactive Learning System is a software program, learning system, and patented heart rhythm monitor developed by Doc Childre, the founder of HeartMath.

HeartMath research has shown that emotions are reflected in a person's heart rhythm patterns. These patterns are transmitted from the heart to the higher brain centers and have powerful effects on the way the brain processes information. Heart rate variability (HRV) is a measure of the naturally occurring beat-to-beat changes in heart rate.

The analysis of HRV, or heart rhythms, is viewed as a powerful, non-invasive measure of neurocardiac function which reflects heart-brain interactions and autonomic nervous system dynamics. One way to record heart rhythms is from pulse wave recordings using a sensor placed at the fingertip or earlobe. This method is used in the Freeze-Framer Interactive Learning System.

The basic idea behind Freeze-Framer is to prevent, manage, and reverse the negative effects of stress. The individual learns to intentionally shift to a positive emotional state. These positive shifts, which benefit both the mind and the body, can be viewed immediately on a computer screen.

According to its website, some of the benefits of Freeze-Framer include the following: increased concentration, improved listening ability, clearer thinking, and improved problem solving skills. Parents also reported calming and balancing effects with children.

Contact information:

Institute of HeartMath
14700 West Park Ave.
Boulder Creek, CA 95006
Phone: (831) 338-8500
E-mail: info@heartmath.org
www.heartmath.org
www.heartmath.org/freezeframer

Hemoencephalographic (HEG) Biofeedback or HEG Neurofeedback

Hemoencephalography (HEG) is the study of blood flow in the brain. More specifically, it is the study of voluntarily controlled oxygenation or blood flow in specifically chosen sections of the brain. It appears that blood flow is poor in certain areas of the brain in people who suffer from various types of conditions including ADHD, autism, stroke, depression, and schizophrenia.

HEG biofeedback was developed in 1994 by Dr. Hershel Toomim, who discovered that he could measure and teach individuals to control the amount of oxygenated blood flowing in the prefrontal lobes using infrared spectroscopy technologies. Dr. Toomim discovered that a person can learn to accomplish this self-regulating skill by applying biofeedback principles. However, unlike EEG neurofeedback, no electrodes are involved.

In many forms of biofeedback and neurofeedback, relaxation is vitally important in the self-regulation training. In contrast, in HEG training, relaxation is not as important as intention and thinking.

Through the use of HEG neurofeedback the blood flow in the prefrontal lobes of the brain is increased. This is accomplished by using an infrared sensor that is positioned in the middle of the forehead. The feedback teaches the individual to exercise his or her frontal lobes. The prefrontal area of the brain is critical in making executive decisions, as well as in focusing attention and memory. The idea is that using HEG biofeedback initially, followed with EEG neurofeedback, may shorten the number of neurofeedback sessions needed as well as possibly improving the success rate.

Contact information:

Biocomp Research Institute
6542 Hayes Drive
Los Angeles, CA 90048
Phone: (800) 246-3526
E-mail: hershel@biocompresearch.org
www.biocompresearch.org
www.adhd-biofeedback.com/HEG.html

Color Therapy or Esogetic Colorpuncture Therapy™

Esogetic colorpuncture therapy™ (ECT) uses light to heal. The idea behind this therapy is that light is actually the medium by which cells in the body communicate and that light is at the core of many body functions. In a colorpuncture treatment, the illuminated tip of an acu-light pen instrument is placed at selected acupressure points on the skin. The acu-light is a small, handheld instrument with interchangeable colored-glass tips which emit incandescent light. It is a non-invasive and extremely gentle process.

In contrast to the use of needles in acupuncture, ECT restores cellular communication by introducing vibrational information in the body through different colored light frequencies via the body's acupuncture meridians. As a result, stability and balance are re-established in the body.

This new method of wholistic healing was developed by Peter Mandel, a German naturopath and acupuncturist. Colorpuncture therapy is done in conjunction with Kirlian photography. Developed in the 1930s, Kirlian energy-field photography makes the electro-magnetic fields surrounding human beings visible. Because the right and left sides of the brain tend to send electrical micro pulses to the opposite sides of the body by way of the nervous system, it is possible to see a visual representation of this brain activity by looking at a Kirlian photograph. Due to the abundance of nerve endings in the fingers, our electro-magnetic field is especially strong around our hands.

Subtle changes in the body's energy states are carefully tracked by means of Kirlian photographs taken before and after treatment. The colorpuncture or light treatments are specifically focused on correcting imbalances revealed by the photographs. ECT has been used in the treatment of a variety of conditions, including ADHD or learning disorders, migraines, and childhood insomnia.

Contact information:

Institute for Esogetic Colorpuncture
1705 14th Street, Suite 198
Boulder, CO 80302
Phone: (303) 443-1666
E-mail: manohar@colorpuncture.com
www.colorpuncture.com

Craniosacral or Cranial Sacral Therapy

Craniosacral therapy involves gentle, non-invasive manipulative techniques which assist the body in its own natural healing. The cranio-sacral system includes all the bones of the skull or head (cranium), face and mouth, extending by a system of hydraulics and membranes to the lower end of the spine or sacrum (tailbone).

The practitioner or therapist listens to the body through palpation (touch), using the bones of the skull and spinal column as handles to manipulate the surrounding skin as well as promoting optimal cerebrospinal fluid flow through the nervous system. Practitioners also work with fascia, loosening adhesions and eliciting emotions attached to stored trauma or ingrained body patterns.

There is a pulse, or rhythm, created by the pumping of the cerebrospinal fluid (CSF), which surrounds and protects the brain and spinal cord. All of the nerves in the human body originate somewhere along this path from the brain down the spinal column.

Throughout the body, the bones are in continual motion as the fluid is pumped. The craniosacral rhythm is detected through hands-on touching. A particular bone may have a non-normal movement; this indicates there is a restriction in the flow of CSF. The practitioner is trained to detect these tiny variations in movement as well as to perform techniques that will open the flow. The aim is to identify and release any restrictions in the body, therefore restoring the free flow of vitality and normal healthy functioning to every part of the body and to the person as a whole.

Dr. John Upledger is generally credited for developing the healing modality of Cranial Sacral Therapy (CST). The gentleness of CST makes it suitable for all ages, from newborns to the elderly. CST has been used in treating various conditions including the following: ADHD, autism, headaches/migraines, chronic back or neck pain, TMJ, insomnia, fatigue, anxiety/depression, and birth trauma.

Contact information:

The Upledger Institute, Inc.
11211 Prosperity Farms Road, Suite D-325
Palm Beach Gardens, FL 33410
Phone: (561) 622-4334

E-mail: edsrv@upledger.com
www.upledger.com

Bach Flower Essences or Oral Flower Essences

Bach flower essences or oral flower essences are a form of complementary medicine sometimes classified as homeopathy and sometimes as herbal medicine. The Bach flower remedies were developed in the 1930s by Dr. Edward Bach, a British physician, bacteriologist, homeopath, and researcher. Since he believed that attitude plays a key role in maintaining health and recovering from illness, Dr. Bach identified 38 basic negative states of mind and created a plant or flower-based remedy for each.

The remedies are derived from non-poisonous plants, shrubs, and trees. They are prepared either by heating the flowers with sunlight in spring water or by boiling twigs and flowers to extract the healing essence.

The human brain is a powerhouse of energy. As individuals, we generate heat, which is energy. Additionally, there is a magnetic field or aura around our bodies. Numerous healing approaches around the world, with the exception of Western orthodox medicine, acknowledge and utilize the basic concept that human beings are essentially energetic beings. Energy fields can change, depending on an individual's physical, mental, or spiritual health. Therefore, choosing or administering Bach remedies needs to be a positive activity, undertaken with loving intent. In this way, positive energy is accompanying the remedies themselves.

Administration in ADHD is typically by mouth. A couple of drops of each remedy required are taken from the bottle and diluted in spring water, or filtered water, or even juice if the child will not drink anything else. Several doses per day will likely be needed. The flower essences are more effective if not taken with food. Sometimes drops are directly applied under the tongue; however, this is often less palatable for most children. The remedies should be stored away from heat, light, and extreme cold, as well as sources of radiation and microwave ovens.

Contact information:

The Bach Centre
Mount Vernon, Baker's Lane
Brightwell-cum-Sotwell, Oxon, OX10 0PZ, UK

Phone: 00 44 (0) 1491 834678
E-mail: centre@bachcentre.com

Flower Essence Society
P.O. Box 459
Nevada City, CA 95959
Phone: (800) 736-9222
E-mail: mail@flowersociety.org

www.bachcentre.com
www.bachflower.com
www.hpathy.com
www.flowersociety.org

BrainTrain Cognitive Training

BrainTrain was founded in 1989 by Joseph A. Sandford, Ph.D., to distribute a cognitive software package entitled the Captain's Log Cognitive Training System. The Captain's Log®, which has since been revised, contains 35 multi-level "brain-training" exercises designed to help develop and remediate such skills as visual and auditory attention, concentration, short-term and working memory, visual-motor coordination, problem solving/reasoning skills, self-esteem, and self-control.

Other software programs available from BrainTrain are SoundSmart® and SmartDriver®. Attention Coach®, one of the modules in SoundSmart, provides drill and practice in following spoken instructions. According to a published brochure, this particular module is used with ADHD children to improve self-control and to develop the ability to maintain attention through multi-step verbal instructions. SmartDriver is described as a visual attention builder. Played like a video game, a child wins by paying careful attention and following the rules of the road.

Although the information on its website clearly states that cognitive training with any of these software modules is not a cure for ADHD, BrainTrain believes its software tools are best used within a comprehensive training program. BrainTrain's software is used in therapeutic, school, and home settings in all 50 states and in more than 20 foreign countries. Additionally, a report on the website indicated that the Captain's Log Cognitive Training Program will be evaluated for its effectiveness in helping to improve the academic performance of school-age children in a three-year study. Dr. David Rabiner (identified in the research section in various chapters throughout this book) will be directing this study funded by the United States Department of Education.

Contact information:

BrainTrain
727 Twin Ridge Lane
Richmond, VA 23235
Phone: (800) 822-0538
E-mail: info@braintrain.com
www.braintrain.com

The Tomatis® Method

The Tomatis® Method was developed approximately 50 years ago by Dr. Alfred Tomatis, a French ear, nose, and throat specialist. Briefly, the Tomatis method is a sensory integration method that uses sound stimulation to develop and improve listening. Some of its basic tenets are as follows: (1) the ear integrates all the sensory information the body receives, (2) the brain receives most of its sensory input from the inner ear, (3) if the ear does not function properly, the brain cannot send the appropriate instructions to the body, and (4) the voice can only produce what the ear perceives. The Tomatis program combines using one's voice and a specially patented headphone that incorporates air and bone conduction sound transmissions with listening to music that is filtered and gated through a device known as the "electronic ear."

The electronic ear, a unique device developed by Dr. Tomatis in the 1950s, makes the implementation of the Tomatis effect possible. The device is connected to a sound source, which is either a CD player or a microphone. The electronic ear acts on this sound and transmits it to a special set of headphones. These headphones allow the individual who wears them to experience sound through both air and bone conductions.

The Tomatis method involves listening sessions, called intensives, which last for several days, with a break period between intensives. Clients listen primarily to audiocassette tapes with pre-programmed sounds of classical music, such as Mozart and Gregorian chants, as well as the child's mother's voice.

By stimulating the brain via the auditory nerve and bone conduction, improvements can be made in such areas as memory, attention and concentration, visual-spatial skills, and communication skills. This method has been used with children with ADHD, dyslexia, autism, Asperger's, and learning problems.

Contact information:

www.tomatis.com—Provides links to Tomatis Centers

Bio-Acoustical Utilization Device (BAUD)

The Bio-Acoustical Utilization Device (BAUD) is a machine that creates sound waves which simulate brain frequencies. Its technology is based on the idea of brain entrainment, using acoustical tones. Dr. G. Frank Lawlis pioneered this technology.

The BAUD uses earbuds or headphones which are connected to the small handheld BAUD device. The unit has adjustments on it that allow for different frequencies to be chosen by the user. It has the flexibility to generate the same frequency or different frequencies on the left and right sides of the brain. This is important, as generally speaking, the left side of the brain tends to perform better with a little faster frequency than the right side. To operate the BAUD, your child simply turns it on and listens to the pulsating sounds.

Finding the correct frequencies for the desired effect is a little more difficult. While it is possible for your child to try various frequencies until he or she finds the one which works the best, it is much better to obtain some guidance. The best way to do this is by working with an EEG neurofeedback provider. The EEG neurofeedback provider will be able to display your child's brainwave patterns on a screen which will allow for specific frequencies that need to be enhanced to be selected. Once this is done, the BAUD unit is programmed to generate the exact frequencies most beneficial for your child.

After the appropriate frequencies are determined, it appears the unit can then be used by itself without further follow-up by the EEG neurofeedback provider. However, there is some evidence that if this unit is used in conjunction with EEG neurofeedback, a synergistic effect may produce quicker and better results. Also if you continue to work with an EEG neurofeedback provider, this professional should be able to make periodic changes to the BAUD frequencies to ensure optimal results. The chapter on EEG neurofeedback has information on how to find an EEG neurofeedback provider for your area.

Contact information:

BAUD Energetics, Corp.
1690 Lawlis Lane
Sanger, TX 76266
Phone: (940) 458-2814
E-mail: info@baudenergetics.com
www.bioacoustical.com
www.theaddanswer.com

Magnetic Therapy

Magnetic energy is the strongest natural force in the universe and the power of magnets is one of the most basic powers of nature. The use of magnetic therapy for health and well-being has an ancient history dating back several thousands of years. Paracelsus, who was born in 1493 in Switzerland and is often considered to be the father of modern medicine, believed that the human body's "life force" was most influenced by the force found in magnets. While millions of individuals in many countries around the world believe in the benefits of magnets and continue to use magnetic therapy, no one really knows how or why magnets appear to help various conditions, including some children with ADHD.

Magnetic products come in several forms, including pillows, mattress pads, comforters, necklaces, medallions or disks, and shoe insoles. In his book *The ADD Answer: How to Help Your Child Now*, Dr. Frank Lawlis discusses magnet therapies in one of his chapters. He indicates that he has been told multiple levels of magnetic stimulation provide the most effective results; he goes on to mention the use of magnetic disks worn on the chest under clothing during the day and magnets inside mattress pads and comforters while sleeping at night. Although various companies sell magnets, Dr. Lawlis mentions that the products of a company called Nikken have been frequently recommended while interviewing various physicians.

Contact information:

www.nikken.com

End Notes

Introduction

1. National Resource Center on AD/HD. Frequently asked questions, pp. 1-12. Retrieved March 23, 2005, from http://www.help4adhd.org.faqs.cfm

2. American Psychiatric Association. (2000). *Diagnostic and statistical manual of mental disorders* (4th ed., Rev. text). Washington, D.C.: Author.

Chapter 1: Being an Informed Parent

1. Jensen, P.S., Martin, D., & Cantrell, D.P. (1997). Comorbidity in ADHD: Implications for research, practice, and DSM-V. *Journal of the American Academy of Child and Adolescent Psychiatry, 36*(8), 1065-1079.

2. CHADD Fact Sheet #3: Evidence-based medication management for children and adolescents with ADHD, pp. 1-12. Retrieved February 23, 2005, from http://www.chadd.org/fs/fs3.htm

3. Barkley, R.A. (2000). *Taking charge of ADHD: The complete, authoritative guide for parents.* (Rev. ed.). New York: The Guilford Press.

4. International Consensus Statement on ADHD (2002, January). Retrieved February 23, 2005, from http://addwarehouse.com/shopsite_sc/store/html/consensus.html

5. Rabiner, D. (2001, October). New treatment guidelines for ADHD from the American Academy of Pediatrics. *Attention Research Update 46*, 1-8. Retrieved February 22, 2005, from http://www.helpforadd.com/2001/october.htm

6. Parker, H.C. It's about time: Promising practices for children and adolescents with ADHD, pp. 1-6. Retrieved February 22, 2005, from http://addwarehouse.com/shopsite_sc/store/html/article10.html

7. Stevens, L.J. (2000). *12 effective ways to help your ADD/ADHD child: Drug-free alternatives for attention-deficit disorders.* New York: Avery

8. Rabiner, D. (2001, October). New treatment guidelines for ADHD from the American Academy of Pediatrics. *Attention Research Update 46*, 1-8. Retrieved February 22, 2005, from http://www.helpforadd.com/2001/october.htm

9. CHADD Fact Sheet #3: Evidence-based medication management for children and adolescents with ADHD, pp. 1-12. Retrieved February 23, 2005, from http://www.chadd.org/fs/fs3.htm

10. Rabiner, D. (2005). *Maximizing the benefits of stimulant medication treatment for children with AD/HD.* Report requested from *Attention Research Update* newsletter at http://wwwhelpforadd.com

11. Vitiella, B., Severe, J.B., Greenhill, L.L., Arnold, L.E., Abikoff, H.B., Bukstein, O.G., Elliott, G.R., Hechtman, L. Jensen, P.S., Hinshaw, S.P., March, J.S., Newcorn, J.H., Swanson, J.M., & Cantwell, D.P. (2001). Methylphenidate dosage for children with ADHD over time under controlled conditions: Lessons from the MTA. *Journal of the American Academy of Child and Adolescent Psychiatry, 40*(2), 188-196.

12. Rabiner, D. (2005). *Maximizing the benefits of stimulant medication treatment for children with AD/HD.* Report requested from *Attention Research Update* newsletter at http://wwwhelpforadd.com

13. National Institute of Mental Health (NIMH). (Rev.2003). *Attention deficit hyperactivity disorder.* Retrieved March 22, 2005, from http://www.nimh.nih.gov/publicat/adhd.cfm

14. Call-Schmidt, T., & Maharaj, G. (2004). Using nonpharmacological treatments in conjunction with stimulant medications for children with ADHD. *Journal of Pediatric Health Care, 18*(5), 255-259.

15. Call-Schmidt, T., & Maharaj, G. (2004). Using nonpharmacological treatments in Conjunction with stimulant medications for children with ADHD. *Journal of Pediatric Health Care, 18*(5), 255-259.

16. CHADD Support: Locate the CHADD chapter nearest you. Retrieved March 23, 2005, from http://www.chadd.org/findchap.cfm

Chapter 2: EEG Neurofeedback

1. Rossiter, T.R., & LaVaque, T.J. (1995). A comparison of EEG biofeed-back and psychostimulants in treating attention deficit/hyperactivity disorders. *Journal of Neurotherapy, 1*, 48-59.

2. Linden, M., Habib, T., & Radojevic, V. (1996). A controlled study of the effects of EEG biofeedback on cognition and behavior of children with attention deficit disorder and learning disabilities. *Biofeedback & Self-Regulation, 21*(1), 35-49.

3. Monastra, V.J., Monastra, D.M., & George, S. (2002). The effects of stimulant therapy, EEG biofeedback, and parenting style on the primary symptoms of attention-deficit/hyperactivity disorder. *Applied Psychophysiology and Biofeedback, 27*(4), 231-249.

4. Fuchs, T., Birbaumer, N., Lutzenberger, W, Gruzelier, J.H., & Kaiser, J. (2003). Neurofeedback treatment for attention-deficit/hyperactivity disorder in children: A comparison with methylphenidate. *Applied Psychophysiology and Biofeedback, 28*(1), 1-12.

5. CHADD Fact Sheet #6: Assessing complementary and controversial interventions, pp. 1-14. Retrieved February 2, 2005, from http://www.chadd.org/fs/fs6.htm

6. About us: Company background. Retrieved February 3, 2005, from http://www.playattention.com

7. Ashton, T. (2001, Spring). Improving attention, reducing behavior problems, and bolstering self-esteem: The many benefits of play attention. *Journal of Special Education Technology, 16*(2). Retrieved February 2, 2005, from http://www.playattention.com/press/ashton.htm

8. Ashton, T. (2001, Spring). Improving attention, reducing behavior problems, and bolstering self-esteem: The many benefits of play attention. *Journal of Special Education Technology, 16*(2). Retrieved February 2, 2005, from http://www.playattention.com/press/ashton.htm

9. Siglin, J. A. (2000). Play attention—focusing on success. *Intervention in School & Clinic, 36*(2), 122-125. Retrieved February 7, 2005, from Academic Search Premier database.

10. Ashton, T. (2001, Spring). Improving attention, reducing behavior problems, and bolstering self-esteem: The many benefits of play attention. *Journal of Special Education Technology, 16*(2). Retrieved February 2, 2005, from http://www.playattention.com/press/ashton.htm

11. NASA Scientific and Technical Information: Spinoff 2003 A real attention-getter. Retrieved February 8, 2005, from http://www.sti.nasa.gov/tto/spinoff2003/hm_2.html

12. Kwan, G. (2002, Spring). Play attention! Can custom-made video games help kids with attention deficit disorder? *Berkley Medical Journal.* Retrieved February 7, 2005, from http://www.ocf.berkeley.edu/~issues/spring02/ADDplay.html

13. Kwan, G. (2002, Spring). Play attention! Can custom-made video games help kids with attention deficit disorder? *Berkley Medical Journal.* Retrieved February 7, 2005, from http://www.ocf.berkeley.edu/~issues/spring02/ADDplay.html

14. BusinessWeek online. (June 14, 2004). My therapist is a joystick: Beneficial games, for everything from phobias to ADHD, are starting to catch on. Retrieved February 3, 2005, from http://cyberlearningtechnology.com/cyber/news.htm

Chapter 3: Interactive Metronome

1. Rabiner, D. (2002, September). Effects of interactive metronome rhythmicity treatment on children with ADHD. *Attention Research Update 57,* 4-7. Retrieved March 1, 2005, from http://www.helpforadd.com/2002/september.htm

2. Special Kids Today. The beat goes on: Interactive metronome helps children with attention difficulties get on track. Retrieved February 2, 2005, from http://www.specialkidstoday.com/resources/articles.thebeat.htm

3. Shaffer, R.J., Jacokes, L.E., Cassily, J.F., Greenspan, S.I., Tuchman, R.F., & Stemmer, P.J. (2001). Effect of interactive metronome treatment on children with AD/HD. *The American Journal of Occupational Therapy*, *55*, 155-162.

4. Interactive Metronome-Clinicians ADHD: IM certification requirements. Retrieved March 24, 2005, from http://interactivemetronome.com

5. High/Scope Education Research Foundation. Timing in child development. Retrieved February 2, 2005, from http://www.highscope.org/Research/TimingPaper/timingstudy.htm

6. Shaffer, R.J., Jacokes, L.E., Cassily, J.F., Greenspan, S.I., Tuchman, R.F., & Stemmer, P.J. (2001). Effect of interactive metronome treatment on children with AD/HD. *The American Journal of Occupational Therapy*, *55*, 155-162.

7. Rabiner, D. (2002, September). Effects of interactive metronome rhythmicity treatment on children with ADHD. Attention Research Update 57, 4-7. Retrieved March 1, 2005, from http://www.helpforadd.com/2002/september.htm

8. Rabiner, D. (2002, September). Effects of interactive metronome rhythmicity treatment on children with ADHD. Attention Research Update 57, 4-7. Retrieved March 1, 2005, from http://www.helpforadd.com/2002/september.htm

9. CHADD Fact Sheet #6: Assessing complementary and controversial interventions, pp. 1-14. Retrieved February 2, 2005, from http://chadd.org/fs/fs6.htm

10. Interactive Metronome. Studies underway or in development with independent agencies. Retrieved February 1, 2005, from http://interactivemetronome.com/im/links.asp?lk=2

11. Special Kids Today. The beat goes on: Interactive metronome helps children with attention difficulties get on track. Retrieved February 2, 2005, from http://www.specialkidstoday.com/resources/articles.thebeat.htm

Chapter 4: Light and Sound Therapies

1. Carter, J. L., & Russell, H.L. (1993). A pilot investigation of auditory and visual entrainment of brain wave activity in learning disabled boys. *Texas Researcher, 4*, 65-73.

2. Joyce, M., & Siever, D. (2000). Audio-visual entrainment program as a treatment for behavior disorders in a school setting. *Journal of Neurotherapy, 4*(2), 9-25.

3. Micheletti, L. S. (1999). *The use of auditory and visual stimulation for the treatment of attention deficit hyperactivity disorder in children.* Unpublished doctoral dissertation, University of Houston.

4. Joyce, M. (2001). New Vision School: Report to the Minnesota Department of Education, unpublished.

5. McMurray, J.C. (2004). Auditory binaural beats enhance EEG-measured beta wave activity in individuals with ADHD. *Hemi Sync Journal.* Retrieved June 13, 2005, from www.monroeinstitute.org/members_section/voyagers/voyages/hsj-summer-fall-2004

6. Sornson, R.O. (1999). Using binaural beats to enhance attention. *Hemi Sync Journal.* Retrieved June 13, 2005, from www.monroeinstitute.org/members_section/voyagers/ voyages/hsj-1999-fall-attention

Chapter 5: Chiropractic

1. Giesen, J.M., Center, D.B., & Leach, R.A. (1989). An evaluation of chiropractic manipulation as a treatment of hyperactivity in children. *Journal of Manipulative and Physiological Therapeutics, 12*, 353-363.

2. Bastecki, A.V., Harrison, D.E., & Hass, J.W. (2004). Cervical kyphosis is a possible link to attention-deficit/hyperactivity disorder. *Journal of Manipulative and Physiological Therapeutics, 27*, 525-529.

3. Elster, E. (2003, July). Upper cervical chiropractic care for a nine-year-old male with Tourette syndrome, attention deficit hyperactivity disorder, depression, asthma, insomnia, and headaches: A case report. *Journal of Vertebral Subluxation Research*, 1-11.

4. Goodman, R.J. (n.d.). National Upper Cervical Chiropractic Association. *Attention Deficit Disorder: Case History.* Retrieved July 6, 2005, from www.nucca.com/articles/attention_deficit_disorder.htm

Chapter 6: Massage Therapy

1. All about massage therapy. (n.d.). Retrieved March 14, 2005, from http://www.massagetoday.com/aboutmt

2. All about massage therapy. (n.d.). Retrieved March 14, 2005, from http://www.massagetoday.com/aboutmt

3. Touch research institute celebrates 10th anniversary. (2002, August). *Massage Today, 2* (8). Retrieved March 16, 2005, from http://massagetoday.com/ archives/2002/08/02.html

4. Field, T.M., Quintino, O., Hernandez-Reif, M., & Koslovsky, G. (1998). Adolescents with attention deficit hyperactivity disorder benefit from massage therapy. *Adolescence, 33*, 103-108.

5. Khilnani, S., Field, T, Hernandez-Reif, M., & Schanberg, S. (2003). Massage therapy improves mood and behavior of students with attention-deficit/hyperactivity disorder. *Adolescence, 38*, 623-628.

6. Osborn, K. (June/July 2004). Attention deficit/hyperactivity disorder: Soma brings peace of mind to families. *Massage & Bodywork*, 140-145.

7. Osborn, K. (June/July 2004). Attention deficit/hyperactivity disorder: Soma brings peace of mind to families. *Massage & Bodywork*, 140-145.

8. Osborn, K. (June/July 2004). Attention deficit/hyperactivity disorder: Soma brings peace of mind to families. *Massage & Bodywork*, 140-145.

9. Elmstrom, R. (2003, April). Massage at preschools and schools: Children who massage one another do not fight! *Massage Today, 3*(4). Retrieved

March 14, 2005, from http://www.massagetoday.com/archives/2003/04/04.html

Chapter 7: Acupuncture

1. Becker, S.A. (n.d.). *A ritalin alternative: Acupuncture in the treatment of ADHD.* Retrieved April 28, 2005, from http://www.chinesemedicalpsychiatry.com/articles/article_ritalin.html

Chapter 8: Aromatherapy and Essential Oils

1. Essential Science Publishing (2004). *Essential Oils Desk Reference* (3rd ed.). Orem, UT: Author.

2. Essential Science Publishing (2004). *Essential Oils Desk Reference* (3rd ed.). Orem, UT: Author.

3. Essential Science Publishing (2004). *Essential Oils Desk Reference* (3rd ed.). Orem, UT: Author.

4. Essential Science Publishing (2004). *Essential Oils Desk Reference* (3rd ed.). Orem, UT: Author.

5. AromaWeb: Finding a qualified aromatherapy practitioner, pp. 1-4. Retrieved March 9, 2005, from http://www.aromaweb.com/articles/aromatherapypractitioners.asp

6. Diego, M.A., Jones, N.A., Field, T., Hernandez-Reif, M., Schanberg, S., Kuhn, C., McAdam, V., Galamaga, R., & Galamaga., M. (1998). Aromatherapy positively affects mood, EEG patterns of alertness and math computations. *International Journal of Neuroscience, 96,* 217-224.

7. Friedmann, T.S.(n.d.). *Attention deficit and hyperactivity disorder (ADHD).* Retrieved March 4, 2005, from http://www.3sistersapothecary.com/html/resources/library/adhd.pdf

8. Essential Science Publishing (2004). *Essential Oils Desk Reference* (3rd ed.).Orem, UT: Author.

Chapter 9: Relaxation Training, Meditation, and Yoga

1. Porter, S., & Omizo, M. M. (1984). The effects of group relaxation training/large muscle exercise, and parental involvement on attention to task, impulsivity, and locus of control among hyperactive boys. *The Exceptional Child, 31*(1), 54-62.

2. Klein, S. A., & Deffenbacher, J. L. (1977). Relaxation and exercise for hyperactive impulsive children. *Perceptual and Motor Skills, 45*, 1159-1162.

3. Kratter, J., & Hogan, J.D. (1982). *The use of meditation in the treatment of attention deficit disorder with hyperactivity.* (ERIC Document Reproduction Service No. ED 232787)

4. Harrison, L.J., Manocha, R., & Rubia K. (2004). Sahaja yoga meditation as a family treatment programme for children with attention deficit-hyperactivity disorder. *Clinical Child Psychology and Psychiatry, 9*(4), 479-497.

5. Medical News Today. Yoga: How does yoga work? What kind of class should I choose? Retrieved March 30, 2005, from http://www.medicalnewstoday.com/medicalnews.php?newsid=10886

6. Jensen, P.S., & Kenny, D.T. (2004). The effects of yoga on the attention and behavior of boys with attention-deficit/hyperactivity disorder (ADHD). *Journal of Attention Disorders, 7*, 205-216.

7. Rabiner, D. (2004, July). Is yoga a helpful complementary intervention for ADHD? *Attention Research Update*, 1-3. Retrieved February 1, 2005, from http://www.helpforadd.com/2004/july.htm

Chapter 10: Physical Exercise

1. Hallowell, E.M., & Ratey, J. J. (2005). *Delivered from distraction: Getting the most out of life with attention deficit disorder.* New York: Ballantine Books.

2. Hallowell, E.M., & Ratey, J. J. (2005). *Delivered from distraction: Getting the most out of life with attention deficit disorder.* New York: Ballantine Books.

3. Barkley, R.A. (2000). *Taking charge of ADHD: The complete, authoritative guide for parents.* (Rev. ed.) New York: The Guilford Press.

4. Altman, N. (n.d.). Endorphins Q & A. Retrieved April 22, 2005, from http://www.healingsprings.com/ENDORPHINS.htm

5. Allen, J. (1980, Winter). Jogging can modify disruptive behaviors. *Teaching Exceptional Children*, 66-70.

6. Wendt, M.S. (2000). *The effect of an activity program designed with intense physical exercise on the behavior of ADHD children.* Unpublished doctoral dissertation, State University of New York, Buffalo.

7. Shipman, W. M. (1985). Emotional and behavioral effects of long distance running on children. In M.L. Sachs & G.W. Buffone (Eds.). *Running as therapy: An integrated approach* (pp. 125-137). Lincoln, NE: University of Nebraska Press.

8. Lawlis, F. (2004). *The ADD answer: How to help your child now.* New York: Viking.

9. Sears, W., & Thompson, L. (1998). *The A.D.D. book: New understandings, new approaches to parenting your child.* New York: Little, Brown and Company.

10. Hernandez-Reif, M., Field, T.M., & Thimas, E. (2001). Attention deficit hyperactivity disorder: Benefits from tai chi. *Journal of Bodywork and Movement Therapies, 5*, 120-123.

Chapter 11: Homeopathy

1. Reichenberg-Ullman, J., & Ullman, R. (2000). *Ritalin-free kids: Safe and effective homeopathic medicine for ADHD and other behavioral and learning problems.* (2nd revised ed.). New York: Three Rivers Press.

2. Lamont, J. (1997). Homeopathic treatment of attention deficit hyperactivity disorder: A controlled study. *British Homeopathic Journal, 86,* 196-200.

3. Frei, H., & Thurneysen, A. (2001). Treatment for hyperactive children: Homeopathy and methylphenidate compared in a family setting. *British Homeopathic Journal, 90*(4), 183-188.

4. Reichenberg-Ullman, J., & Ullman, R. (2000). *Ritalin-free kids: Safe and effective homeopathic medicine for ADHD and other behavioral and learning problems.* (2nd revised ed.). New York: Three Rivers Press.

Chapter 12: Essential Nutrients as Supplements

1. Stevens, L. J. (2000). *12 effective ways to help your ADD/ADHD child: Drug-free alternative for attention-deficit disorders.* New York: Avery.

2. Harding, K.L., Judah, R.D., & Gant, C.E. (2003). Outcome-based comparison of Ritalin® versus food-supplement treated children with AD/HD. *Alternative Medicine Review, 8,* 319-330.

Iron

1. Sever, Y., Ashkenazi, A., Tyano, S., & Weizman, A. (1997). Iron treatment in children with attention deficit hyperactivity disorder: A preliminary report. *Neuropsychobiology, 35,* 178-180.

2. Konofal, E., Lecendreux, M., Arnulf, I., & Mouren, M. (2004). Iron deficiency in children with attention-deficit/hyperactivity disorder. *Archives of Pediatrics & Adolescent Medicine, 158*(12), 1113-1115.

Magnesium

1. Kozielec, T., & Starobrat-Hermelin, B. (1997). Assessment of magnesium levels in children with attention deficit hyperactivity disorder (ADHD). *Magnesium Research, 10*(2), 143-148.

2. Starobrat-Hermelin, B., & Kozielec, T. (1997). The effects of magnesium physiological supplementation on hyperactivity in children with attention deficit hyperactivity disorder (ADHD): Positive response to magnesium oral loading test. *Magnesium Research, 10*(2), 149-156.

3. Rabiner, D. (1999, June). Magnesium supplementation as a treatment for ADHD. *Attention Research Update*, 8-9. Retrieved March 7, 2005, from http://www.helpforadd.com/yr1999/june.htm

Zinc

1. Bekaroglu, M., Aslan, Y., Gedik, Y., Deger, O., Mocan, H., Erduran, E., & Karahan, C. (1996). Relationships between serum free fatty acids and zinc, and attention deficit hyperactivity disorder: A research note. *Journal of Child Psychology and Psychiatry, 37*, 225-227.

2. Akhondzadeh, S., Mohammadi, M., & Khademi, M. (2004). Zinc sulfate as an adjunct to methylphenidate for the treatment of attention deficit hyperactivity disorder in children: A double blind and randomized trial. *BioMed Central Psychiatry, 4*, Retrieved June 29, 2005, from http://www.pubmedcentral.nih.gov/articlerender.fcgi?tool=pubmed&pubmedid=15070418

3. Bilici, M., Yildirim, F., Kandil, S., Bekaroglu, M., Yildirmis, S., Deger, O, Ulgen, M., Yidiran, A., & Aksu, H. (2004). Double-blind, placebo-controlled study of zinc sulfate in the treatment of attention deficit hyperactivity disorder. *Progress in Neuro-Psychopharmacology & Biological Psychiatry, 28*, 181-190.

4. Rabiner, D. (2004, March). A double-blind, placebo-controlled study of zinc sulfate as a treatment for ADHD. *Attention Research Update*, 1-3. Retrieved March 7, 2005, from http://www.helpforadd.com/2004/march.htm

Essential Fatty Acids

1. Stevens, L.J., Zentall, S.S., Abate, M.L., Kuczek, T., & Burgess, J.R. (1996). Omega-3 fatty acids in boys with behavior, learning, and health problems. *Physiology & Behavior, 59* (4/5), 915-920.

2. Aman, M.G., Mitchell, E.A., & Turbott, S.H. (1987). The effects of essential fatty acid supplementation by Efamol in hyperactive children. *Journal of Abnormal Child Psychology, 15* (1), 75-90.

3. Richardson, A.J. (2004). Clinical trials of fatty acid treatment in ADHD, dyslexia, dyspraxia and the autistic spectrum. *Prostaglandins, Leukotrienes and Essential Fatty Acids, 70*, 383-390.

4. Richardson, A.J., & Puri. B.K. (2002). A randomized double-blind, placebo-controlled study of the effects of supplementation with highly unsaturated fatty acids on ADHD-related symptoms in children with specific learning difficulties, *Progress in Neuro-Psychopharmacology and Biological Psychiatry, 26*(2), 233-239.

5. Rabiner, D. (2002, June). The effect of fatty acid supplementation on ADHD symptoms. *Attention Research Update*, 2-4. Retrieved March 7, 2005, from http://www.helpforadd.com/2002/june.htm

6. Richardson, A.J., & Montgomery, P. (2005). The Oxford-Durham study: A randomized, controlled trial of dietary supplementation with fatty acids in children with developmental coordination disorder. *Pediatrics, 115*(5), 1360-1366.

7. Rabiner, D. (2005, June). Fatty acid supplementation helps children's academics and behavior. *Attention Research Update*, 1-4. Retrieved June 27, 2005, from http://www.helpforadd.com/2005/june.htm

8. Stevens, L., Zhang, W., Peck, L., Kuczek, T., Grevstad, N., Mahon, A., Zentall, S.S., Arnold, L.E., & Burgess, J.R. (2003). EFA supplementation in children with inattention, hyperactivity, and other disruptive behaviors. *Lipids, 38*(10), 1007-1021.

Glyconutrients

1. Dykman, K.D., & Dykman, R.A. (1998). Effect of nutritional supplements on attentional-deficit hyperactivity disorder. *Integrative Physiological and Behavioral Science, 33*, 49-60.

North American Ginseng & Ginkgo Biloba

1. Lyon, M.R., Cline, J.C., Totosy de Zepetnek, J., Shan, J.J., Pang, P., & Benishin, C. (2001). Effect of the herbal extract combination Panax quinquefolium and Ginkgo biloba on attention-deficit hyperactivity disorder: A pilot study. *Journal of Psychiatry & Neuroscience, 26* (3), 221-228.

L-Carnitine

1. Van Oudheusden, L.J., & Scholte, H.R (2002). Efficacy of carnitine in the treatment of children with attention-deficit hyperactivity disorder. *Prostaglandins, Leukotrienes and Essential Fatty Acids, 67*(1), 33-38.

Vitamin Therapy

1. Haslam, R. H.A. (1992). Is there a role for megavitamin therapy in the treatment of attention deficit hyperactivity disorder? *Advances in Neurology, 58*, 303-310.

Chapter 13: Dietary Changes and Food Sensitivities

1. Studies show that diet may trigger adverse behavior in children: HHS urged to recommend dietary changes as initial treatment. (1999, October 25). *CSPI Newsroom.*

2. Schab, D.W., & Trinh, N. (2004). Do artificial food colors promote hyperactivity in children with hyperactive syndromes? A meta-analysis of double-blind placebo-controlled trials. *Journal of Developmental & Behavioral Pediatrics, 25*(6), 423-434.

3. Rabiner, D. (2005, April). Dietary intervention for ADHD: A meta-analysis. *Attention Research Update,*1-3. Retrieved July 12, 2005, from http://www.helpforadd.com/2005/april.htm

Chapter 14: Environmental Factors

1. Taylor, A.F., Kuo, F.E., & Sullivan, W.C. (2001). Coping with ADD: The surprising connection to green play settings. *Environment and Behavior, 33*, 54-77.

2. Kuo, F.E., & Taylor, A.F. (2004). A potential natural treatment for attention-deficit/hyperactivity disorder: Evidence from a national study. *American Journal of Public Health, 94*(9), 1580-1586.

Glossary of Assessment Instruments and Research Terms

Attention Deficit Disorders Evaluation Scale (ADDES)

The ADDES enables educators, school and private psychologists, pediatricians, and other medical personnel to evaluate and diagnose ADHD in children and youth from input provided by primary observers of the child's behavior. There is a school version, which is a reporting form for educators, and a home version, which is a reporting form for parents.

Attention Quotient (AQ)

Attention Quotient scores are based on equal measures of visual and auditory vigilance, focus, and speed. Vigilance is a measure of inattention as shown by two different types of errors of omission. Focus reflects the variability of mental processing speed for all correct responses. Speed reflects the average reaction time for all correct responses and helps identify attention processing problems related to slow mental processing.

Attention Endurance Test (AET)

This assessment of attention basically requires children to perform a clerical paper and pencil task where careful attention to detail is necessary to obtain a good score.

Auditory Sequential Memory subtest of the Illinois Test of Psycholinguistic Abilities (ITPA)

The ITPA in an individually administered test for children aged 4 to 8, measuring 12 functions employed in the acquisition and use of language. The test consists of 10 main subtests, one of which measures Auditory Sequential Memory.

Burks' Behavior Rating Scale (BBRS)

The BBRS includes 110 items, each describing a behavior not frequently observed in normal children. A parent or teacher indicates, on a 5-point response scale, how often the behavior is seen in the child being evaluated.

Conners' Continuous Performance Test (CPT)

The CPT is a computerized test which is widely used in ADHD research and clinical assessments for individuals aged 6 or older. Response patterns provide information that allows the practitioner to better understand the type of deficits that might be present. For example, some response patterns suggest inattentiveness or impulsivity, while other response patterns may indicate activation/arousal problems or difficulties maintaining vigilance. This test lasts for approximately 14 minutes; children with ADHD have a difficult time maintaining attention for the entire time period.

Conners' Rating Scales

The CRS is an instrument that uses observer ratings and self-report ratings to help assess ADHD and evaluate problem behavior in children and adolescents. There are three versions: parent, teacher and adolescent self-report. All of these versions have a short and long form available. These various versions allow flexibility in collecting varying perspectives on a child's behavior from parents, teachers, caregivers, and the child or adolescent.

Various versions or subtests appear in the research studies cited throughout this book. Among them are the following: Conners' Abbreviated Parent-Teacher Questionnaire, Conners' Teacher Rating Scale, Conners' Short Form Parent Rating Scale, IOWA-Conners' Behavior Rating Scale, Conners' Global Index, and Conners' Hyperactivity Scale

Control Group

This is a group, similar to the treatment group, which does not receive the treatment so it can be compared to the treatment group.

Disruptive Behavior Disorders (DBD) Rating Scale

The DBD Rating Scale can be used to assist in diagnosing ADHD, Oppositional Defiant Disorder, or Conduct Disorder. Teachers and parents complete the scale by rating a child on 45 items in regard to the frequency or degree of displaying behaviors, such as "often interrupts or intrudes on others" or "often fidgets with hands or feet or squirms in seat."

DuPaul Parent Ratings of ADHD

This 18-item rating scale is used for diagnosing ADHD in children and adolescents and for assessing treatment response. It is directly linked to DSM-IV diagnostic criteria and comes in two formats: a parent questionnaire assessing home behaviors and a teacher questionnaire evaluating classroom behaviors.

Fruit Distraction Test (FDT)

The FDT measures the child's ability to selectively attend to relevant information. The child is asked to name a series of colors as quickly as possible. These colors are presented on cards, and some are surrounded by irrelevant and distracting images.

Integrated Visual and Auditory Continuous Performance Test (IVA CPT)

IVA is a combined auditory and visual continuous performance test designed to help the clinician make an accurate diagnosis of ADHD for individuals ages 6 through adult. It provides information to help differentiate between the four sub-types of ADHD—ADHD predominantly inattentive, ADHD predominantly hyperactive-impulsive, ADHD combined, and ADHD not otherwise specified. Scores are divided into four categories: attention, response control, attribute and symptomatic.

Matching Familiar Figures Test (MFFT)

The MFFT measures both attention to visual detail and impulsivity. It requires selecting the appropriate matching picture from among six possibilities. One of the possibilities is an exact match while the other five are slightly different in one detail each. The responses are timed.

Nowicki-Strickland Locus of Control Scale (LCS)

The LCS, which consists of 40 yes-no questions, measures the degree to which children believe that reinforcement is a result of their own behavior (internal locus of control) or a result of fate or chance (external locus of control). Scores can range from 0 (internal locus of control) to 40 (external locus of control). High scores on the LCS correlate negatively with achievement.

Peabody Picture Vocabulary Test (PPVT)

The PPVT is an oral test of receptive (listening) vocabulary. It is given individually and not timed, although it typically takes only 15 to 20 minutes to administer.

Placebo

This is a "fake" treatment given to one group of participants while the treatment being tested is given to another group. The "placebo effect" is a phenomenon in which a fake treatment can sometimes improve a person's condition simply because the individual expects that it will be beneficial. To separate out this factor and some other variables from a treatment's true benefits, placebo-controlled studies are often used. If those individuals on the new treatment fared significantly better than those who took the placebo, the results will help support the conclusion that the treatment is effective.

Raven Coloured Progressive Matrices

This test consists of 36 problems with matrices detailed in a colored background. It is internationally recognized as a culture-fair test of nonverbal intelligence, designed for use with children between the ages of 5½ and 11½. The child is required to select a missing figure through analogy reasoning to complete a matrix-like arrangement.

Response Control Quotient (RCQ)

RCQ scores are derived from visual and auditory prudence, consistency and stamina scales. Prudence measures impulsivity and response inhibition as shown by three different types of errors of commission. Consistency is a measure of general reliability and variability of response times and is used to measure the ability to stay on task. The stamina score is used to identify problems related to sustaining attention and effort over time.

Slosson Oral Reading Test—Revised (SORT-R)

The SORT-R is a screening test of word recognition that can be used with regular education populations and also with most special populations. It gives a brief measure of reading ability and is most useful in identifying those with reading disabilities.

Test of Variables of Attention (TOVA)

This is a computerized visual continuous performance test that measures errors of omission, errors of commission, average response time for the correct responses, and the standard deviation of the response time for correct responses. These four variables are interpreted as measures of inattentiveness, impulsivity or failure to inhibit response, speed of information processing, and variability in attention. Since the TOVA is computer administered and scored, it provides objective data that is relatively bias free.

Treatment Group

This is the group given the treatment or treatments being tested.

Wechsler Intelligence Scale for Children-Revised (WISC-R)

The WISC-R is a general test of intelligence that is a collection of 13 distinct subtests divided into two scales, verbal and performance. It is designed for children ages 6 to 16. Verbal, performance, and full scale scores are calculated.

Werry-Weiss-Peters Activity Scale (WWPAS)

The WWPAS provides a way of assessing the activity level of a child in specific situations, such as doing homework, watching television, eating meals, and playing.

Wide Range Achievement Test-Revised

The WRAT-R contains three subtests: reading (recognizing and naming letters and words), spelling (writing symbols, names, and words), and math (solving oral problems and written computations). It is designed to measure school codes needed to learn the basic skills of reading, spelling, and math, rather than comprehension, reasoning, and judgmental processes.

Woodcock-Johnson (WJ-R) Tests of Cognitive Ability

This battery of tests, which can assess specific strengths and weaknesses, measures such factors as short-term memory, processing speed, auditory processing, and visual processing. It takes approximately 60 to 70 minutes to administer. The battery has various scales including verbal ability, thinking ability, cognitive efficiency, predicted achievement, and general intellectual ability.

Information about Authors

LaVonne Kirkpatrick, Ed. D.

With over 30 years teaching experience, Dr. LaVonne Kirkpatrick has taught courses dealing with various teacher preparation issues, including ADHD. She has presented at state, national, and international conferences. She has also been principal investigator of a school-based grant which involved working with ADHD children and their families.

Her interest in helping young children learn and be successful began over 30 years ago when she became an elementary classroom teacher. While teaching elementary school, she had her first experiences working directly with ADD/ADHD children and their families. This interest and connection has continued to the present day as an assistant professor in the College of Education and Health Professions at the University of Arkansas.

As a faculty member, Dr. Kirkpatrick teaches elementary majors who are preparing to become classroom teachers. She has supervised numerous student teachers, as well as working directly with their mentors teachers in the field. With such close contact, she has heard novice and experienced teachers alike voicing their concerns over trying to reach all of the children they're teaching. She has witnessed firsthand their struggles in dealing with the ADD/ADHD children in their classrooms. Often their frustration in not feeling confident or not knowing where to turn next is expressed. Principals and guidance counselors, as support personnel, are also seeking answers. Parents of these children are at a loss as well.

Through all of these experiences, Dr. Kirkpatrick's desire to help ADD/ADHD children has only grown stronger. She began seriously focusing on researching information about viable treatment options approximately eight years ago. This book is the result of her strong commitment and desire to assist ADD/ADHD children and their families which has spanned over three decades.

Rick Kirkpatrick, M.S.W., L.C.S.W.

Rick Kirkpatrick has provided mental health counseling to children and adults for a variety of conditions, including ADD/ADHD, in both private practice and in various mental health facilities for approximately 15 years. He has presented at both state and international conferences on the utilization of "alternative therapies" for ADD/ADHD and other mental health conditions.

As Director of the Integrative Health and Therapies Program at a rehabilitation hospital, one of his responsibilities was to research complementary and alternative treatment options. Those showing a high level of validity were integrated into the traditional therapies that were provided for patients. Mr. Kirkpatrick observed that combining traditional medicine with various non-traditional therapies often resulted in improvements that neither treatment approach could produce on its own. He took this same integrated approach in the treatment of ADD/ADHD, resulting in improving the lives of both children and adults who suffer from this condition.

The authors now wish to share what they have learned with the general public. It is their hope that *The ADD/ADHD Revolution* will be of assistance in helping those who suffer from ADD/ADHD have a better and more rewarding life.

Index

978-0-595-36935-5
0-595-36935-9